DEWEY

To A Great Baseball Fan!

DEWEY

BEHIND THE GOLD GLOVE

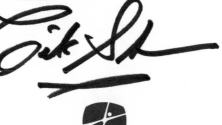

DWIGHT EVANS
WITH ERIK SHERMAN

TRIUMPH
BOOKS

Library of Congress Cataloging-in-Publication Data available upon request.

This book is available in quantity at special discounts for your group or organization. For further information, contact:

Triumph Books LLC
814 North Franklin Street
Chicago, Illinois 60610
(312) 337-0747
www.triumphbooks.com

Printed in U.S.A.
ISBN: 978-1-63727-565-8
Design by Nord Compo

This book is dedicated to Susan,
my beloved wife of 53 years

In loving memory of my boys,
Timothy and Justin

CONTENTS

FOREWORD

WHEN DWIGHT EVANS came up to the Red Sox as a 20-year-old rookie at the end of the 1972 season, I could see he had talent both offensively and defensively—*especially* defensively. And even though I was playing in my 12th major league season and was 12 years older than Dwight, we quickly became close because we had a lot in common.

First and foremost, though, I think Dwight and I hit it off as well as we did because we understood how tough a game baseball is to play—and that we both had to work hard to become good players.

The success that Dwight and I had in baseball certainly didn't come easily. But we were always there for one another when needed. I can remember sitting with Dwight in Fenway Park or in another stadium on the road when one of us was struggling at the plate and how we talked about hitting over and over again. We just tried to help each other get through slumps. And that's what friendship and being good teammates is all about.

We played together in what many believe to be the greatest World Series of all time in 1975. In Game 6, Dwight made a leaping catch in front of the right-field fence at Fenway that meant a lot to his career. We all knew on the Red Sox how good he was in the outfield, but now the rest of the baseball world did too. The catch alone was great, but the fact that he had the presence of mind to throw the ball back to first to double up the baserunner made it even more impressive. I was playing first base, and one of my initial thoughts was how not too many other outfielders would have had the instincts to make that throw. Of course, the Fenway fans erupted in cheers. The fans in Boston were always great and on our side. As players, we knew that, and it helped us tremendously.

Almost from the very beginning of Dwight's career, he had serious family challenges caring for his two sons afflicted by Neurofibromatosis. That had to have been very tough for him, but he rarely talked about it. That was a part of his life he kept inside.

Occasionally, he would mention to me how he spent the night in the hospital with one of his sons or when one of them was going in for surgery. I always thought that for Dwight to be able to handle those problems, he had to be a strong, strong person. I don't know how he managed it all and still played the game as well as he did. The game is tough enough without going through everything he did with his boys.

Dwight would play in the second-most games in the history of the Red Sox. I think that says it all because I know all the games I played in, and it wasn't easy. So, for him to be the second all-time really says a lot.

I lost my son, Michael, in 2004 and Dwight would lose his sons, Timothy and Justin, in more recent years. Sadly, this is another thing we now have in common. And because I knew what I went through after losing my son, I had a sense of what Dwight was feeling when he lost both of his. So, I tried my best to give him the support he needed. Because that's what friends do.

Dwight is one of the mentally toughest people I've ever met. I can't believe how strong he is. I wouldn't have been able to handle losing two sons like he has. Dwight has always been such a positive, special person. And for as great a competitor as Dwight was, that trait was always matched by the kind of man he is.

—Carl Yastrzemski
1989 Baseball Hall of Fame inductee
Triple Crown winner, 1967
18-time All-Star

PREFACE

I FIRST ENTERTAINED THE IDEA OF WRITING an autobiography several years ago after my pastor, Dan Betzer—who knew a little something about writing books, with more than 20 of his own—planted the seed in my head. As a former All-Star right fielder for the Boston Red Sox and a father who helped raise two very sick boys who would eventually succumb to complications from Neurofibromatosis, it was a story I felt needed to be told.

It was important to me to convey that while I may have been a professional ballplayer, I'm just an imperfect human being who has, along with my wife and children, lived through a humbling life of great family adversity, tragedy, and sorrow. Of course, we are hardly alone with our struggles, so my hope is that this book will inspire others going through similar difficult times and reassure them that there is still a life that we must carry on with.

I believe setting an example on how to conduct oneself during troublesome times is so important. After the death of my two sons, a lot of people approached my wife and me, asking variations of, "You've got to be mad at God, right?" But we're not, because we believe in the hereafter and that we will see our boys again. I believe you can be a regular guy like I am and still have faith. I think that's why the beautiful poem "Footprints in the Sand" sizes up my walk on this earth perfectly. I'm never alone, as God is with me always through the good times and the bad times.

I also have so many wonderful memories from my life in baseball to tell. As I knew the book would need to be a delicate balance between baseball and my personal life, I prayed about finding the right coauthor to collaborate with me. And every answer pointed to Erik Sherman, who interviewed me for a poignant book on the '86 Red Sox seven years ago. I've always been a very personal and quiet individual but felt comfortable opening up to him. I don't generally like talking about myself, so his ability to get me to open my heart the way he did and bring out stories I hadn't thought about in so many years was impressive. Sherman's baseball knowledge, recall, and researching ability kept me in check regarding the most minute details of games and events from decades ago. We actually made a game out of his recollection versus mine on specific players and feats from the past over the course of the project. Thankfully, for a correct answer I had about a Rick Burleson play, I avoided getting shut out!

Erik also interviewed some of my Red Sox teammates like Jimmy Rice, Freddie Lynn, Bill Lee, Marty Barrett, and Bruce Hurst—all great players in their own right—to come up with anecdotes of my time with them that we could discuss for the book. Erik handled that so well and then to hear what they told him—how much they cared and what my being their friend and teammate meant to them—was very humbling to me. Because you never know what impact you've made on people, to hear what they said was very special. And their stories also acted to trigger some wonderful memories that I tell in this book. Due to my family issues during my playing days, I didn't always have the ability to enjoy the exceptional moments like I wish I could have. But working on this project and hearing what others said reminded me of some of the things I missed.

After the seemingly countless hours of reflection and discussion with Erik I did for this book, I came to realize some of the things I miss the most from my days as a ballplayer. First and foremost, I loved playing before the incredibly passionate Red Sox fans at Fenway Park. And to be able to play as long as I did in front of those fans was a special treat. Another thing I long for is the competition between me and the pitcher. To have that feeling of being at the plate and battling with the game on the line—especially at Fenway—was a dream come true. I loved and thrived on the big moments. When you're out of baseball, you don't think about those things. But working on this book brought me back to what it felt like to play this great game again.

On a more personal level, Erik helped me remember things that I had conveniently forgotten—including very difficult topics surrounding the boys—and memories I really didn't want to rehash. But again, if they can help somebody going through similar circumstances, that was the best reason to include them in the book.

I'm proud of what I've accomplished in my 50-year involvement in professional baseball. And I still love being involved in the game. In my current role with the Red Sox in player development, I can still relate to today's ballplayer and talk to them in a way that builds them up. And I think that's so important. The game is so negative. If you *fail* as a hitter 70 percent of the time, you're considered a great player. And you can hit four bullets in a game and still go 0-for-4. That makes it hard to stay positive. So, for six weeks in spring training and periodic visits throughout the season, I'm all about building players up and keeping them in as positive a mode as you can have in this game.

And for Red Sox fans who cheered me on and supported me throughout my 19 seasons in Boston, it makes me feel good they will, at last, have a full picture of a regular guy who happens to have a strong faith that got him through some highly trying times in his life. They may have watched me play six months a year, but they never knew who I truly was or what I was going through. Now they'll have their chance to find out.

—Dwight Evans
Fort Myers, Florida
April 2024

INTRODUCTION

O N A LATE JULY AFTERNOON IN 2017 while I was working on the manuscript for my book, *Two Sides of Glory*, about the 1986 Red Sox, I received an email from Dwight "Dewey" Evans. We had tried for months to set up an interview for the project, though Dwight's time had been consumed with caring for his oldest son, Timothy, who was battling stage-four brain cancer stemming from his lifelong battle with Neurofibromatosis (NF)—the same disease that also afflicted his youngest son, Justin. "We'll make it happen," he assured me in the email. "And thank you for your prayers. We take that very seriously." His manner told me all I needed to know about his high character. I thought, *Who else treats people with so much kindness and respect while dealing with such intense family trauma?* Dwight would then, amid everything going on in his personal life, somehow find the time to meet with me at Fenway Park later that summer and help make my chapter about him one of the most poignant in the book.

Tragically, Dwight and his wife, Susan, would lose both of their sons—Justin on Easter Sunday 2019, and Timothy just 10 months later—from the effects of NF. Their daughter, Kirstin, mercifully healthy her entire life, was now their sole remaining child. As a father myself, I couldn't fathom the hurt Dwight was going through at that time. And as an author of baseball books that chronicle players who deal with great challenges in their lives, it was another reminder to me of how celebrated athletes often face the same suffering and pain as everyday people.

In spring 2021, I recalled Dwight telling me during our interview four years earlier how his pastor in Florida suggested he write a book. "I've got a bunch of stories," he told me then. "My wife says, 'You should write them down.' But I don't think of them unless someone talks to me about them." *An autobiography by an all-time-great Red Sox slugger with a Gold Glove and rifle arm would stand alone as a wonderful story*, I thought. But when you add everything he and his family endured throughout almost his entire illustrious career, I believed it would be a fascinating and, in many ways, inspiring book. So, I wrote Dwight a letter expressing those thoughts and hoping that the timing would be right for him to collaborate on his memoir. Shortly thereafter, Dwight called me to confirm he was ready to go, but told me I would need to be his "Dick Bresciani"—the late longtime Red Sox public relations man with an aptitude for remembering the most minute baseball-related details—to assist in his recall of long-ago events. I told Dwight those were big shoes to fill, but that I would do my best.

Our initial meeting for the project was at a restaurant on Market Street in Lynnfield, a suburb of Boston. I arrived first and waited out front. Moments later, out in the distance, I saw Dwight and Susan—walking together hand-in-hand. Two things struck me right away. The first was how youthful this married couple of more than 51 years appeared. And the second was how jovial and ebullient they both seemed. After all, within the space of just the previous two years, they had been through so much sorrow with the passings of their sons. Once in the restaurant, when I had a private moment with Susan at our table, I said, "I'm so impressed with how you both carry yourselves the way you do. I would have been broken if I lost one or both of my children. How do you stay so upbeat?" Susan smiled and didn't hesitate, asking me earnestly, "Erik, what kind of witnesses [to God] would we be if we *didn't* stay upbeat?" I knew right then and there I was in the presence of two of the most mentally strong individuals I had ever known.

Of course, anyone who watched baseball during the 1970s and 1980s already knew about Dewey's *physical* strength by his stature, tape-measure home runs, and gifted throwing arm. But what some may not have realized was how he often played through immense pain from sciatic nerve problems and bone spurs and endured bouts of vertigo brought on by vicious beanball incidents that may well have ended the careers of other players. Yet, through all the extreme personal and professional challenges he faced, at the time of his retirement, he found himself on the Mount Rushmore of legendary Red Sox outfielders with Ted Williams, Carl Yastrzemski, and Jim Rice.

In fact, what's most remarkable is how Dewey was the rarest of ballplayers who actually *improved* with age—having a markedly better second half of his career than his first. He was already a 12-year veteran when, starting in 1984 and running through 1989, he *averaged* 102 RBIs a season. And nobody hit more home runs in the American League or had more extra-base hits in all of baseball during the decade of the '80s than Evans did. Yet, when discussing this book project with baseball fans, the first thing they bring to light is not Dwight's big offensive numbers, but rather his special right arm that was like kryptonite to baserunners and helped earn him eight Gold Glove Awards.

There were signature moments in his career, too—perhaps none greater than his outstanding catch in right field in the fabled Game 6 of the 1975 World Series—one which Reds Hall of Fame manager Sparky Anderson called the *greatest* he ever saw. The brighter the spotlight, the better he played—as his .300 batting average, three home runs, three doubles, one triple, and 14 RBIs in the '75 and '86 World Series combined would attest to.

Yet, his storied career remains an enigma in many respects. Dwight, with all his humility, would never think, say, or write this himself—so I will. He is one of the most *underrated* outstanding players in the history of baseball. First, he didn't get Hall of Fame voting love from the sportswriters when eligible, and then, in recent years, when the Contemporary Baseball Era Committee was formed to consider candidates who played the prime of their careers largely in the 1980s—he absurdly wasn't even on their 2022 ballot of eight players. This was particularly strange since Evans was nearly voted into the Hall of Fame by the Modern Baseball Era Committee in 2019, falling just four votes shy of the 12 needed for induction.

It's also a conundrum to me why his No. 24 is still in circulation with the Red Sox. Retiring numbers has always been a "feel" kind of thing, and that certainly should apply to Evans, whose style of play embodied what the Red Sox mean to their millions of fans. And he put up the numbers. Dewey's total number of games played for the club is second only to Yastrzemski, and he's ranked fourth in total hits, extra-base hits, and doubles, and fifth in home runs and RBIs. In each of those categories, every Sox player ranked above him is a Hall of Famer. Combine all this with his superb defensive play, the courage and character he exemplified off the field, and his 46 years in the organization, and this honor should be a no-brainer for a club that embraces its history like Boston does.

Perhaps the reason why his greatness is often overlooked can be explained this way. For as elite a ballplayer as Dewey was, he largely avoided the media and was often overshadowed by larger-than-life teammates like Yaz, Rice, Carlton Fisk, Fred Lynn, and Wade Boggs. He was also humble to the point where he would hit a three-run homer but give most of the credit to the two guys who got on base in front of him. Evans simply preferred to forego the limelight after games in order to get home to his family—a noble quality, but not a recipe to market oneself as the star he was.

But these are exactly the reasons why this intimately told story is so special. For the first time, the publicity-shy and private Dwight Evans opens his heart to you—the fan and the reader—in revealing a life with the extreme highs and lows of a Shakespearean drama. At its core, this is a book about an iconic Red Sox player whose internal fortitude, courage, and faith sustained him through the trials and tribulations surrounding the diagnosis, treatment, and deaths of two sons tragically afflicted with NF, and still performed at the highest levels of his sport for two decades.

His example should serve as an inspiration to us all.

—Erik Sherman
New Rochelle, New York

CHAPTER 1

A PRIVATE MATTER

JIMMY RICE NEVER KNEW. The teammate and friend with whom I shared the Fenway Park outfield for 16 seasons never knew how neurofibromatosis (NF), a genetic disorder of the nervous system that causes tumors to grow on nerves, had devastated the lives of my two sons, Timothy and Justin, throughout most of my Red Sox career and beyond. But Jimmy's unawareness of their severe condition would change on an early July evening in 2006 up in a Legends Suite at Fenway Park, where Rice and I were hosting a group of 25 fans as team ambassadors for the Red Sox. Earlier in the day, Jimmy and I had attended the 20th Annual NF Golf Tournament at the International in Bolton, Massachusetts. My wife, Susan, and I had just been named honorary chairs of the event that year, and Jimmy read a bio about my family and the immense challenges we had endured for more than three decades in a pamphlet distributed at the tournament. Upon learning further details of our struggles from me at the suite, one of the most physically imposing men in baseball history became overwhelmed with emotion.

"Dewey! Dewey! I never knew! I never knew!" he kept repeating as tears welled up in his eyes. "I just *never* knew this was going on with your kids. I had no clue!" That reaction from a big, strong guy like Jimmy Rice kind of took me back. I was really touched

1

by his sensitivity and concern. It would be natural to wonder how a teammate of mine for all those years could have been so uninformed about my sons' serious malady. But the fact is it was entirely my doing. None of my teammates, except for my closest friend, confidante, and mentor in baseball, Carl Yastrzemski—who suffered the pain of losing his own son, Michael, 20 years ago— really knew any of the details or the severity of the situation. In baseball, you talk about the game; you talk about the weather. Nobody wants to hear about your problems. You just don't share all that much about your family life.

Freddie Lynn, who manned centerfield so magnificently for us in Boston for seven seasons, would say how he and some of our teammates knew my boys were not well—the disfiguring effects of the disease were very evident—but they didn't know specifically the term for what they had or the extent of how serious it was. They also didn't want to intrude, so they respected our privacy. Bill Lee, our masterful left-handed pitcher for so many years, would say he felt a sense of helplessness; the typically loquacious "Spaceman" simply didn't know what to say to me. And I get it. It's the kind of thing where you're not sure how to ask and what to ask about it. Neurofibromatosis is a word a lot of people can't even pronounce. And when you've got 30 or so guys in the clubhouse—not counting coaches, players on the disabled list, and clubhouse workers— there's a lot going on. It's all business in there. So it was never discussed, even when Susan and I would bring the boys and our daughter, Kirstin, to the Red Sox clubhouse. On such occasions, we acted as if nothing was wrong, and the boys behaved like happy and healthy kids. Susan and I didn't do anything other than just love them and try to treat them as normally as possible. One thing you didn't want to do was make them feel sorry for themselves.

As for me, I never made any excuses about how my lack of sleep and worrying about my family may have affected my play on the field. There were many nights I was at Fenway Park after having come straight from the hospital following one of my boys' many surgeries and wasn't having a good game. And you know what? I just had to eat it. I had to eat if from the press. And I even had to eat it from the fans. But the thing that I did find out after 19 years of playing in Boston was how passionate New England fans are. If you're playing poorly, they're going to boo you. If you make a great play, they're jumping up and down, screaming, and cheering you on. It's not that they're fickle—they're just emotional. And I love that about them.

I remember my former Red Sox teammate Rick "the Rooster" Burleson telling me after we traded him to the Angels, "I miss New England fans because, in Anaheim, if I dive and make a great play in the hole at short, you've got twenty thousand people just saying 'Wow.' But in Boston, the reaction would just be off the charts after a play like that." What's sad is that I see some players who come to the Red Sox who either just don't get that or don't have the make-up to play in Boston. It can be a tough place to play, but once you've been accepted by Red Sox fans, you're accepted for life.

The ballpark would become like a sanctuary for me. Once I drove into that Fenway parking lot, it was like a free zone where I could leave everything else behind. And the longer I played, the more it became a refuge where I could release my anxieties and stress for a few hours. But once I left the ballpark, there 'it' was again—that *thing* that would jump on me when I would often stop by the hospital and stay there as long as I could—then go home and try to grab a little sleep before coming back out the next day and doing it all over again.

In the early years after the diagnosis of both of my sons, I didn't handle things as well as I did later on. I probably "wore it" too much on the outside. They always say public speakers are 10 times more nervous on the inside than they appear on the outside. That's not what I was like early on. I couldn't easily contain my feelings, and it affected my play. Certain people would say things about my performance, but they didn't know what I was going through at home. I don't know how they would have handled it if they knew, but thankfully I played long enough where I could eventually rise above the criticisms and excel at a high level for many years in the big leagues.

After nearly two decades playing with the Red Sox—a period that including winning eight Gold Gloves, leading the American League in home runs and all of baseball in extra-base hits during the '80s, and being a part of two pennant-winning teams—then another 24 years in the organization after my career ended, Boston is as big a part of me as anything else in my life.

I've come a long way since the days of walking barefoot wearing shorts and a T-shirt to Kailua Elementary School in Hawaii.

CHAPTER 2

GROWING UP QUICKLY

MY EARLY CHILDHOOD YEARS were a weird and confusing—yet still, at times, enjoyable—period in my life. I was born in Santa Monica, California, moved to Kailua, Hawaii, at eight months old, and then transferred between these two picturesque states several times for the first 10 years of my life. The transition of changing schools so frequently was unsettling for me. I was always "the new kid" growing up.

Still, living in Hawaii as a youngster, when we did, certainly had its perks. It was the kind of place where my siblings and I did our homework on the beach and, while my two older brothers surfed, I skim-boarded. I was small at that time and the surf boards were so big I couldn't handle them. But with skim boards, just as the tide started going out a bit and the water level was barely above the sand, you jumped on one and rode it for about 20 feet until you hit a little wave and did a flip into the water. I also had my first exposure to baseball—albeit by myself. There was a high school ballpark right across the street from our house and I would bring a ball and a bat and spend hours hitting the ball down the length of the field and back. So, Hawaii was great fun and would have been a wonderful place to stay.

But stability was not a choice for my family, as my father, Duff, worked for Sheraton hotels, which, in 1959, acquired four hotels on Waikiki Beach in Honolulu that were owned by Matson, a Pacific Ocean shipping services company. When my parents, four siblings, and I moved back to California from Hawaii for the last time, it was on one of the Matson Lines cruise ships—free of charge—because my father was working for the company. We were such brats on that trip. We'd play shuffleboard and fire those shuffle discs off the side of the ship. From that point on, the cruise staff understandably kept a close eye on us.

Arriving in California, we settled in Northridge in the San Fernando Valley. Entering yet another school, this time at age 10, wasn't easy, and I was frequently getting into fights. After living in sunny Hawaii, my skin had gotten very dark. Because of this, instead of calling me Dwight, some of my classmates called me "Da' Black." Well, those were "hooking" words for me. I don't know why them calling me "Da' Black" upset me so much, other than it just wasn't my name. And I would hook in a second if I got riled. As I moved on to junior high school, I became even more of a fighter, often taking my bouts behind a handball court where other kids would stand around and watch. In all my years fighting as a young person, I only lost one fight. I was just eight years old, and this older kid popped me good a couple of times— just dropping me. Despite the advice my father always gave me about fighting—jab two or three times and then follow with a right hook—this older kid's head went back, but then he looked at me with an expression that said, *Okay, you little punk—take this!* Pow! Pow! He just smoked me.

Thank goodness I found baseball. I was the only one in my family interested in the game. Out of all of them, my older brother, Duff, certainly could have played, as he had a great arm and could throw the ball further than I could at that time. But his primary interests were surfing with my other older brother, David, and his '57 Chevy, where he was frequently found underneath making repairs and putting on loud mufflers. David was the prototypical surfer dude in the groovy '60s. So it was often my mother, Marie, who would play catch with me in our backyard. My father did at times, too, but often it would be with his shirt and tie on with the car running before he was off traveling for his sales job at Sheraton. His greatest contribution to my playing ball was introducing me to one of his dear friends, Pinky Woods. Woods had pitched for the Hollywood Stars, a Triple-A team, after spending three years hurling for the Red Sox during World War II. It was always a treat when he would come by and play catch. He must have done a good job teaching me a few things, because my third-grade teacher, Miss Reed, took notice. We were playing softball in recess one time and, after watching me for a while, she said, "You should play little league." But there was just one problem—little league cost $20 to join, money our family didn't have to spend on such things. But we always had food on the table and my mother could make leftovers out of anything, though feeding a large family like ours meant staying within a budget.

That's when a very special and influential man in my life—my grandfather, David Lionel Evans—saved the day. He was a dentist who started his business in Beverly Hills and then moved it to the San Fernando Valley, where he had a five-acre ranch four miles from where we lived. He had every type of tree you could imagine—trees that grew oranges, peaches, tangerines, avocados, and almonds—and would board horses there as well. I went to him and told him what the situation was, and he said, "If you plow my fields in between the trees where the weeds grow, I will give you the twenty dollars you need to play ball." I was ecstatic. For a 10-year-old, driving a tractor was like driving a Ferrari! I worked hard, but it was fun work. True to his word, when I finished plowing the fields, he gave me $20, and I went and put that down at Northridge Little League and got my Indians uniform.

My grandfather and I became even closer than we were because of baseball. He would take me to my little league games and sit in a fold-up chair with an umbrella, watching them all. Afterward, I would be filthy with dirt all over me, but it never stopped him from taking me in his Thunderbird to an A&W Root Beer restaurant, where we would sit and talk about the game while having hamburgers and root beer. He died of lung cancer in 1968, just a few years before my Major League career began. Out of everyone in our family, I wish that he had lived to see me play for the Red Sox. That would have meant so much to both of us.

As a 10-year-old, I was a pitcher and third baseman—positions I played until I entered professional baseball. I was fortunate to have as my first little league coach a great guy named Chet Randolph. As a fireman, he had more free time than most of the other coaches and would throw batting practice for as long as you needed him.

A couple of years later, I made the Northridge Little League All-Star team and really learned how to play the game. We went to the regional playoffs but fell a couple of rounds short of becoming eligible to play in the Little League World Series in Williamsport, Pennsylvania.

From there, I made the All-Star teams in the Pony League and then the Colt League while also playing high school ball. But because of districting, I was going to Granada Hills High School at the time. I made the '67 junior varsity team, but only as an alternate, because the coach had all the Granada Hills players that had gone to the Little League World Series in 1963 starting over everyone else on the club. The only opportunities I really had to play were in practice games against the varsity team, where I would hit home runs and drive balls all over the field. But during most of our JV regular season games, I had to sit on the bench dressed in my school clothes and couldn't play. I was put on what Eddie Kasko, my first manager with the Red Sox, would call "KP Duty." When someone asked him what KP Duty was, he said, "Can't Play." So that's kind of like what I was on—KP Duty—in the 10th grade.

Despite being on KP Duty, things were looking up at age 15, as I would meet the love of my life, Susan, at a house party. I had no lines whatsoever. I pretty much just walked up to her and asked if she wanted to see *The Graduate*. She said yes despite thinking, at the time, that I was a pompous and arrogant guy because of how quiet and shy I was.

During the movie, in my efforts to be all cool and snuggle with Susan, my big move was to put my arm around her. But I royally messed that up—I accidentally *elbowed* her right in the forehead! I nearly knocked Susan out as she saw stars, but she forgave me enough to go out to Bob's Big Boy Restaurant after the movie, where we shared a hamburger with little chopped onions cut in half, an order of fries with blue cheese dressing, and two lemon Cokes. Our first date was salvaged!

As for the dire baseball situation, that would resolve itself the following year when I went to live with my grandparents and transferred to Chatsworth High School, which was seven miles from Granada Hills High School. I made the varsity team as a junior, played both third base and pitcher, and was named to the All-West (San Fernando) Valley Team. I was a standout for Chatsworth Varsity just a year after not even being given the chance to prove myself in Granada Hills.

As a senior, I had a 6–0 pitching record to go along with a .552 batting average, and the *Van Nuys News Press*, our local paper, dubbed me "Mr. Everything" for my two-way playing ability. I was also named the Most Valuable Player in the West (San Fernando)

Valley League, which was a very big honor considering how that part of California was a breeding ground for some truly outstanding ballplayers. During the 1969 high school season, I played against future big-league stars like Gary Matthews from San Fernando Valley High and Doug DeCinces from James Monroe, as well as Robin Yount's older brother, Larry, a pitcher at nearby Taft. In fact, the competition was so strong in that area that DeCinces, who played in the same Colt and Pony Leagues when I did, didn't even get drafted by a big-league team out of high school. Despite all his talent, he had to wait until he was playing at Los Angeles Pierce College in Woodland Hills before the San Diego Padres came calling. With the Los Angeles area so large and the climate so nice, it was a hotbed for producing big league stars. High schools often had winter leagues, too, which allowed young players to improve their skills all year long. The No. 1 draft pick in 1969, the year I graduated high school, was Jeff Burroughs from nearby Long Beach; and two of my future Red Sox teammates, Fred Lynn and Bill Lee, were also raised in the Los Angeles area.

Throughout my senior season, professional scouts were at every game. By mid-June of the 1969 Major League Baseball Amateur Draft period, I heard from 14 teams. The first question they would ask my high school coach, Coach Matula, was whether they should draft me as a pitcher or everyday player. Coach Matula told them he thought I would be a better everyday player. I had a good arm—once striking out fourteen hitters in a seven-inning game—but I didn't know how to pitch. We didn't have pitching coaches in high school to teach me the finer points of the craft. So I had to rely on observing my pitching idols growing up—Sandy Koufax and Don Drysdale of the Dodgers and Juan Marichal of the Giants. But when I would try to throw sidearm like Drysdale, my arm hurt more, so that didn't work out too well. But I did throw enough strikes to get through a game.

Back then, the scouts who were interested in signing you gave you a big index card that had their team's logo on it, and you had to fill it out with your name, address, and phone number. I filled out 14 cards—from the Angels, Cubs, Cardinals, and so on—but never one from the Red Sox. But they must have been watching me, I thought, because I soon got a call from one of their lead scouts who said, "Dwight, I'm Joe Stephenson from the Red Sox. I'd like to come over, meet your parents, and see if we can sign you." We set up a meeting for the next day in my family's living room—my parents sitting on each side of me on a long couch we had. I was six feet tall and weighed 170 pounds at 17 years old, but the scout was probably sizing me up when looking at my father, who was over 6'4", and my mother, who was 5'8", and figured I would end up being bigger than I was.

"Dwight, I was at Dodger Stadium but didn't see you play," Stephenson said, referring to a tournament my high school team had just played in. A little miffed, I asked, "Well, why do you want to sign me then?" And he goes, "Well, I heard from other scouts that you would be a pretty good pick."

I don't know if his next move was a negotiating ploy, but he pulled his chair up to our long coffee table and, after about 45 minutes, said, "Well, I want you to know that the Boston Red Sox want to sign you. And the Boston Red Sox are willing to give you $7,500." At this point, I'm getting elbowed from both my mother and father because we didn't have any money. So, while I'm getting jabbed on both sides, Joe tells me all about the Red Sox and sells me hard on the organization. Then he goes for the close. "So, how do you feel about the offer, Dwight?" And I said, "Well, with all due respect, Mr. Stephenson, I'm not going to sign for that." Joe sat back in his chair, threw his arms back, and gave me a look like I was a little punk before saying, "Well, what's it going to take to sign you?" I said, "I want $10,500 and a college education."

Meanwhile, my parents were pretty much beating me up at this point. But I had it in the back of my mind that a very close friend of my father's was Elroy "Crazy Legs" Hirsch, who was inducted into the Pro Football Hall of Fame in 1967 following a remarkable career as a wide receiver with the Los Angeles Rams. Hirsch was now the athletic director at the University of Wisconsin, and I knew that, as a favor to my dad, I would have a chance at either a partial or full scholarship to play football there. I loved football—especially the contact at the positions I played at as an offensive wide receiver and a defensive back—but baseball was what I really wanted to do. Still, football at Wisconsin was my wild card.

After hearing what it would take to sign me, Joe again threw his arms back and said, "I don't have the authority to sign you for that kind of money, so I'm going to have to call the Boston Red Sox." Joe went back into our kitchen, which was only 20 feet away, to make his call. While he was on the phone, my parents were just bruising my ribs with their elbowing, whispering to me things like, "What are you doing?" I told them, "If they say no to my demands, then I'll go to the University of Wisconsin and play football."

We listened closely to what Stephenson was telling the Red Sox on the other end of the phone and heard the entire conversation from his end. "This guy would be really good to have in our system." "He comes from a good family." "I think he'd be a great fit for us." "I think we really need to sign him."

After 15 minutes, Joe hung up the phone and pulled up his chair again. "I want to tell you something, Dwight," he said. "You're quite the negotiator. The Boston Red Sox just gave me the authority to sign you for $10,500, and they will give you that college education." Now my parents are looking at me like I'm the best thing since sliced bread—hugging the Red Sox fifth-round draft choice from both sides. I felt pretty good about myself when I signed that first professional contract.

Just two days later, I would see Stephenson again—this time at Los Angeles International Airport. He was accompanied by the Red Sox seventh-round draft choice and future big-leaguer Steve Barr. Joe was seeing us both off before we flew out to Jamestown, New York, to begin our professional careers in the New York–Penn League. At just 17 years old, it would be my first trip east of California or away from home. My life would never be the same.

CHAPTER 3

BECOMING DEWEY

TALK ABOUT PECULIAR BEGINNINGS. When I reported for duty to the Jamestown Falcons of the Rookie-Level New York–Penn League, it certainly wasn't what I had envisioned my first exposure to professional baseball to be. The Falcons were on the road for five days and didn't have a uniform for me or their other 15 recent draftees that had just arrived. The club told us to buy a long-sleeve jersey and to bring cleats, and eventually they would have uniforms for us. Because of this situation, we had 16 guys working out in jeans, hats, and shoes. So, I was playing in my jeans and a red jersey, thinking it was the appropriate color since it was a Red Sox farm team. I quickly found out they actually wore blue jerseys. Anyway, that was my outfit, and, during that period, I did well in batting practice. The coaches who stayed in Jamestown took notice. Soon thereafter, they made some player moves and I got my uniform.

The level of young talent on the Falcons was something I had not experienced to that point. I may have been MVP of the West Valley in the San Fernando Valley, but I soon found out we had the MVP of Chicago, the MVP of Dallas, and the MVP of San Francisco, so the ability of these other kids was tremendous. It made me feel pretty small. In fact, even after I got my uniform, I didn't play in a game for another week.

But after hitting a few home runs in batting practice one day, my manager, Jackie Moore, told me, "I'm going to start you at third base tonight." I said, "Great!" and thought this was my big opportunity to shine. There was just one issue. We had a guy named Don Nowlin, a player with limited talent, who had just come back from Vietnam, and the Red Sox had promised him an opportunity to play third base. There was little doubt he was probably thinking how he didn't want to sit on the bench while some 17-year-old punk took his position, and he made his feelings clear. Shortly before that game, Nowlin was fielding grounders at third base while I was taking batting practice. Once I finished hitting, I ran the bases. As I was passing Nowlin at third, I could have sworn he spit at me. I looked up and there wasn't a cloud in the sky, yet, out of the blue, I got sprayed with something. I glanced over at him but didn't really want to tangle with a 23-year-old Vietnam veteran with two tattoos on each arm and sleeves that were cut off showing his big biceps. I had smartened up a little bit from my younger days by not wanting to hook him. But he stayed on me hard during this period—once giving me the finger from the back of the dugout during a game when I was on the field.

It was an especially hard time for me because I was so young. I would cry myself to sleep at night. I didn't have family or any friends around—and I really missed Susan. I was staying in a boarding house and was getting just $5 a day for meal money, which paid for maybe two McDonald's meals and little else back in 1969. But it was Nowlin who was really getting under my skin.

After a week of making the most of my playing time, yet having to endure Nowlin's daily harassment, I went to talk to Moore about it. Jackie calmly reiterated to me that the guy had been in Vietnam and the club wanted to give him a shot. "In fact," Moore said, "we're playing him at third tonight. We promised him we would give him a chance. I've got to see what he can do, but don't worry; you'll be back in there in no time." That night, Nowlin had a big game and would stay hotter than a firecracker over the next three contests, so they couldn't take him out of the lineup. But then an interesting development occurred. The Red Sox's highly touted 1968 second-round draft choice, right fielder Curt Suchan, who was leading the club in every offensive category, badly wrenched one of his knees and had to come out of a game. Moore turned to me on the bench and asked if I could play right field. Although I had never played the position in my life, I emphatically replied, "Yeah! I can play there!" I grabbed my glove and sprinted to right field. I didn't care where they put me as long as I played, and I never left the position. It would mark the beginning of a 23-year run playing right field in professional ball.

———————

After the season with Jamestown ended, I played in the Florida Instructional League that fall with the goal of adapting to the outfield and polishing my overall baseball skills as rapidly as possible. I was extremely fortunate to have coaches like Sam Mele and Frank Malzone.

Mele was a terrific right fielder in the '40s and '50s for several big-league clubs and had managed the Minnesota Twins for seven years—a tenure that included an American League pennant in 1965. He had a real big-league presence about him. He took a liking to me, and I had an attachment to him as well because he truly cared about me and nurtured me, teaching me about playing right field and throwing from the position. I had a good arm, but it was a matter of corralling it and working on using my legs more. And Malzone was a six-time All-Star with the Red Sox during the '50s and '60s and was one of the premier sluggers of his time. I learned a lot about hitting from him. I couldn't have asked for two better mentors and, as a result, the Instructional League really helped to improve my game.

But for as encouraged as I was about my progress as a young baseball player, my heart ached for Susan, and I hated being away from her. I called her every chance I got. When I returned home to California after the Instructional League ended, we spent every moment we could together, and we both realized we couldn't live without one another for another baseball season. So, just before reporting to spring training in March 1970, I decided to ask her to marry me. I would do it the old-fashioned way by going to her father, Harold Severson, first, and asking for his blessing. I was barely 18 and, after staring at him for a moment, I said nervously, "I would like to ask for your daughter's hand in marriage." I knew him well and he was a great guy, but he asked seriously, "How are you going to take care of her?" Of course, he had a point. I was making $500 a month for the six-month period covering the minor league season and the instructional league. So, I was guaranteed to make only $3,000 in baseball over the next year. Still, I was ready with an answer to his question. "Well, I'm hoping to make it in baseball," I told him. "I'm going to give myself four years to make the major leagues. And if I don't make it, we'll come back to California, and I'll become either a fireman or a policeman." At that time, the LAPD was one of the most elite police forces in the country and that appealed to me. And if I became a fireman, I would work 15 days a month and have the rest of it off, which was also enticing. Harold understandably wasn't thrilled, out of concern for his very young daughter's welfare, but he knew this was what Susan and I wanted, and that we were deeply in love, so he was satisfied with my plan and gave his blessing. After proposing to Susan with the engagement ring I bought for her right after my 18th birthday, we quickly set a wedding date for September of that year. We were both so excited about being married that we couldn't wait for my season with Greenville to be over at the end of August.

The Red Sox minor league spring training that year in Ocala, Florida, presented another thrill. The Red Sox brought in this guy who was going to work with us on running for about a week. His name was Jesse Owens. At the time, I only knew a little bit about Owens' history. By 1970, Jesse was 56 years old, but he was still a very striking man with a strong presence both physically and personality-wise. He could still run and enjoyed teaching us how to improve on that skill. Owens took a liking to me and complimented me on my running. It was a neat experience and, as I got older and learned more about history, I watched highlights of Jesse running in Munich at the 1936 Olympics in front of Adolf Hitler. Owens just blew people away, winning four gold medals in the track-and-field competitions. What a great athlete he was, and what an impressive man for me to have worked with. He was certainly one of the truly special people I encountered over my career.

Playing for the Greenville Red Sox in South Carolina was, without question, a better experience than what I had in Jamestown. Not only was it A-Ball, a level higher, but we would win both the first and second halves of the season to claim the 1970 Western Carolinas League title. And thanks in part to the Instructional League, I had a strong season, hitting .276 with seven home runs and 68 RBIs in 108 games.

I also got to play for a manager named Rac Slider, a minor league lifer with a great big-league name. Rac came out of Texas, and I loved the guy. He was only about 5'7" and weighed maybe 160 pounds, but he had that Napoleon Bonaparte attitude—always with a chip on his shoulder. We had a catcher who was around 240 pounds—the biggest player on the team—and Rac stood him up in front of everybody in the clubhouse and squared off with him. Of course, the guy wasn't going to fight Rac because he would have squeezed him in half. But it was Rac's way of letting the team know who was in charge.

The catcher certainly wasn't the only person Rac wanted to make a point with. He even made an example out of me, and, to this day, I have no idea why. During a game that season, I grounded out to end an inning and turned around looking for a teammate to bring me my glove. All of a sudden, I see someone running out to right field. It's Rac! He goes to me in his Texas drawl, "Come on baby, you and me, right over there in the bullpen! Let's go!" So, I walked with him to the bullpen, scratching my head and wondering what was going on. Once we got there, he fired his hat down, faced off with me, and shouted, "Let's go! You throw the first punch!" I said, "I'm not going to hit you, Rac. The next thing I know, I'll get my release papers tomorrow morning." I then kept asking him what I did wrong, but he wouldn't give me an answer, and no punches were thrown. Rac was a tough guy to play for, but he was the kind of guy you respected more after reflecting on how much you learned from him about being a man at just 18 years old. Ironically, I would play for Rac again many years later when he was named the Red Sox bullpen coach in 1987 under John McNamara. He was then promoted to third base coach in 1988 after Joe Morgan took over and remained there through the rest of my time in Boston.

As soon as the season ended in Greenville and right before I had to report for instructional league again in Sarasota, Florida, Susan and I had a quick wedding at a chapel in the canyon of Canoga Park, California. My two grandmothers sat in the front row with my mother, crying their eyes out. My father didn't attend the ceremony because he thought we were too young to get married, telling me it wasn't going to last (53 years later, I am confident in saying his prediction was wrong). So, his not coming was his way of protesting the wedding. Instead, he worked in Madison, Wisconsin, that day. After the ceremony, we had a small reception in Susan's parents' backyard in Chatsworth. We then rushed off for a one-night honeymoon in Newport Beach. We paid $42.10 for our room on the beach, a lot of money for a couple of 18-year-old kids. After a one-night stay at Susan's parents' house, the next morning we got in our car and drove three and a half days from Chatsworth to Sarasota. All we had was $400. We didn't have a phone and could barely afford anything. Susan made her own clothes and, after the season ended, we would paint houses with friends from high school to make extra money. We didn't know any better. We did what we had to do. But we couldn't have been happier.

But as my prospects in baseball were becoming brighter and I was married to the love of my life, the Vietnam War was raging and dividing the country in half—a deep concern of mine at the time. In 1970, I had a high military draft number of 220, so the anxiety of getting selected was real. My view of the war had evolved. When I was 16 years old and in 11th grade in 1968, I remember thinking, *I want to go to Vietnam. I want to support my country.* But the next year, I began seeing guys that I graduated high school with coming back from Vietnam in boxes and remember saying, "I don't think I want to go to Vietnam now." And none of my friends did anymore, either. It was a nasty war fought halfway around the world, and no one even knew why we were fighting. Because I was in the minor leagues right out of high school, I wasn't involved in all the protesting that went on at colleges across the country. But I recall how divisive the war was. While we were told by the government that we were fighting the advancement of communism, which I believed to be important, I kept thinking, *What a place to go and fight.* Sometimes I think we get into wars too easily and maybe stay too long. But I have always loved our military and the spirit of America.

The military would take up to draft number 150, so I was never selected for service, enabling me to report to the Winston-Salem Red Sox of the Class-A Carolina League in the spring of 1971. Don Lock, who had a nice eight-year career as a centerfielder primarily with the Washington Senators in the '60s, was our manager and was fun to play for, respected everybody, and tried to help his players as much as he could to improve their game. Don was a perfect manager for me, teaching me to take the right paths and routes on balls hit to me in right field. He also gave me my nickname, Dewey, which would stick with me for the rest of my life. He started calling me Dewey because we had a pitcher named Don Newhauser whom he already called Newey. And we had a Latin player whom he nicknamed Louie. So, it was Newey, Louie, and Dewey. I liked being called Dewey because I wasn't really happy with my name, Dwight. I don't know why, other than I didn't know of too many other people named Dwight in my lifetime other than Dwight Eisenhower. So, Dewey sounded pretty good to me, and it really stuck.

Poor Susan got her first taste of the travails of being a baseball wife. The wife of one of my teammates, a woman named Bunny, told her one day, "You know, when they get to the major leagues, they all cheat and leave their wives." Susan said, "What? What are you talking about?" So, she came home that night and told me, "Dwight, I don't ever want you to make it in baseball because Bunny told me all the players leave their wives." I had to calm Susan down and reassure her that wouldn't be the case with us.

That season, I started hitting for more power as a 19-year-old, hitting 12 home runs and driving in 63 for Winston-Salem in 118 games. I also played alongside future Red Sox teammates Cecil Cooper and Rick Burleson for the first time and the three of us enjoyed big years. Although the club finished with a .500 record, the season was a great success in terms of the progress I made as a ballplayer. The result was a promotion from A-Ball straight to Triple-A Louisville of the International League, a significant jump as I would skip playing for Double-A Pawtucket.

At Louisville, I was now one step away from the major leagues. But jumping two levels of minor league ball at age twenty was a daunting task and I struggled mightily at the beginning. Even the *Sporting News* picked up on it, writing in April 1972, "He won't make it this year, but Dwight Evans, a rookie outfielder, is considered one of the best prospects in the business by Red Sox executives."

Right around the All-Star break, I was hitting just .172. That's when Louisville Colonels' manager, Darrell Johnson, who would later manage me with the Red Sox, came up to me during a road trip and said, "Dwight, you've got eight games to get your hitting affairs in line. If you don't, I've got to send you down to Pawtucket." I appreciated that fair warning because I really didn't know why I hadn't been sent down earlier, as I was really struggling. But maybe because my defense was as strong as it was, Johnson felt I was still helping out the team.

Once we got back from the road trip a day later, I told Stan Williams, a 35-year-old, 14-year major league veteran pitcher trying to hang on in baseball—and my roommate when we travelled—what Johnson said to me. "Well, if you're going to go down," Williams told me, "you're going to go kicking, fighting, and scratching. You're going to work. Come to the ballpark early tomorrow." So, the next morning, the two of us went to the ballpark and Williams positioned me in front of the concrete right field wall—which was 15 feet high—and started pitching to me. Stan had a rubber arm and threw hard with what we called a "heavy ball." He threw fastballs and curveballs at me for hours. That's how players were back then—helping teammates out and trying to make them better. And Stan helped me out tremendously. He noticed how my left shoulder would come out a little bit when swinging like I wanted to pull the ball and he'd say, "Stay there with your shoulder! Stay there with your shoulder!" again and again. This went on for five days, but I still wasn't hitting a lick during games. But then, finally, on the night of June 13, everything clicked, and I went 4-for-4 against future big league pitcher Jesse Jefferson.

From that point on, I tore up the league by going 42-for-68 (a .618 average)—a streak almost unheard of—which got my batting average up to .240; and then I would hit .400 the rest of the way to finish the season at .300, with 17 home runs, 95 RBIs, and 90 runs scored—good enough to earn me International League MVP honors. *The New York Times* picked up on the story and wrote, "It was one of the greatest batting climbs in International League history." The tremendous finish had me going from the outhouse to the penthouse!

Louisville finished the International League regular season in first place with an 81–63 season. We moved on to the Triple-A playoffs and, after I hit a home run to win one of those games in Toledo over the Mud Hens, Johnson called me into his office to give me the news that every minor leaguer dreams of hearing. "Dwight, you're going to the big club," he said with a smile. "You're going to catch the earliest flight and meet them in New York. And one more thing. You're going to need a sports coat." At just 20 years old, I was now a member of the Boston Red Sox.

CHAPTER 4

BAPTISM BY FIRE

I WAS IN AWE. Getting called up to the major leagues was one thing, but having my first taste of big-league life in the original Yankee Stadium, often referred to then as the "Cathedral of Baseball," took the thrill up another notch. It's where I watched Roger Maris hit his then single-season-record-setting 61st home run on television in 1961. It's where Babe Ruth played. Then you had the red stone monuments of Lou Gehrig, Miller Huggins, and Ruth out in deep left center field. When I arrived there that first day, I was walking on air in that massive outfield, looking up and around that old, historic stadium, thinking, *What am I doing here?* I knew there was a reason for my call-up during the heat of the pennant race, but I just wasn't quite sure what it was at that point, especially with Reggie Smith installed as the Red Sox starting right fielder at that time. But it didn't matter. This was baseball nirvana.

But some of that warm feeling diminished a bit when it was time to take batting practice. There were certain fringe players in their early thirties who didn't play every day. Clinging to their jobs, they saw me as a threat to their livelihood and wouldn't let me stay in the batting cage. When I jumped in to get a few swings, they told me to get out after taking just one. They clearly didn't want me to do well. It was a real dog-eat-dog world.

On September 12, 1972, my first day in the major leagues, the
Red Sox were clinging to a half-game lead over the Yankees and
Baltimore Orioles, and a one-game edge over the Detroit Tigers.
It didn't get much tighter than this. It would also be my first taste
of the longstanding, storied Yankees–Red Sox rivalry that featured
the top two young catchers in the American League—Carlton Fisk
and Thurman Munson. For as talented as they both were, they had
contrasting styles of play and were built very differently from one
another. Carlton was 6'3", weighed 220 pounds, and was a polished
player with a great arm. Pitchers loved throwing to him, and he
controlled the game behind the plate as well as anyone. Fisk was
also a terrific athlete with speed for a catcher. Munson was a pudgy
5'11", 190-pound guy who had a non-athletic, working-class look,
and wasn't the most graceful player, but he was tough as nails
and would eat dirt to win a ballgame. A real gamer and a terrific
hitter, Munson was the AL Rookie of the Year in 1970 and Fisk
won the award in 1972. In the years ahead, until Thurman died in
a plane crash in 1979, they had some issues and a genuine dislike
for one another, which only fueled the rivalry between our teams.

The Yankees would win that game 3–2, beating our ace Luis
Tiant. I didn't appear in that game and would have to wait until a
September 16 contest at Fenway to make my major league debut.
I entered that game as a pinch-runner for Reggie Smith and then
replaced him in right field in the top of the seventh inning. The
Cleveland Indians' very first batter that inning, Tommy McCraw,
hit a line drive into the right-center-field gap. The sun was so
devastating in right field at Fenway before they added the upper
level which blocks it out now. On this play, I fought the sun, laid
out, and made a diving catch to bring the crowd to their feet. It
was my first Fenway Park standing ovation in what would be my
home away from home for the next 19 years and a moment I will
never forget. To this day, I still get goosebumps thinking about it.

The next inning, I had my first big league at-bat and just missed the chance to do something special. Cleveland pitcher Bill Butler threw me a hanging slider that I saw so well, but I just missed it, popping out to shortstop.

I wouldn't have to wait long for my first major league hit. That would come the very next day against future Hall of Famer Gaylord Perry when I came up as a pinch-hitter in the bottom of the ninth inning. The first pitch he threw me looked like a 120-mile-an-hour fastball on the outside corner and I thought, *Oh my gosh, this is the big leagues. How am I going to hit that?* Not knowing Gaylord at that time, there very well may have been a little baby oil or something on that pitch to help it move the way it did. But the next pitch he threw me was a hanging slider that I jumped all over, hitting a line drive so hard off the Green Monster that, as I was rounding first base, the ball was already being thrown into second. So, I had to put on the breaks and slide back into first base and settle for a long single. In any other ballpark, it would have been a sure home run, but I had to settle for a single because of The Wall. The irony is that Gaylord owned me after that, and I didn't get another hit off him for another four years—a very long oh-fer!

My breakout day would come on September 20 in a double-header sweep of the Baltimore Orioles. I had four hits including a triple and my first major league home run off Eddie Watt into the netting above the Green Monster. Our manager Eddie Kasko rewarded me by starting me in left field 16 times down the stretch in our fight for the American League East Division title. It was baptism by fire for this very green rookie. I truly felt the confidence that Eddie instilled in me, though I wasn't comfortable in left field at all.

Many people have the misconception that the outfield is the outfield and that all three positions are played the same way. But that's not the case at all. It's like if you put a great shortstop at third base, he becomes average. He might catch the ball, but he's a great shortstop playing out of position. It's the same thing in the outfield. Left field is as different from center field and right field as shortstop is from second or third base. Before this became common knowledge, Gold Gloves used to be awarded to three outfielders, not to one at each of the three outfield positions. As a result, you would often get two centerfielders and just one corner outfielder winning the award, which was unfair. I was hoping to get moved to right field the following season, and there was already some talk of moving Smith to center field and Tommy Harper to left.

Once I started playing every day, some of the veteran starters and pitchers began giving me the support that I needed to get acclimated to big league life.

My bond with Carl Yastrzemski began right away. From our earliest days as teammates, we would go out to dinner after games and fish on his boat during the off-season. What a lot of people don't understand about Carl is that he is a private person who doesn't let too many people in. And he's always been a deeply personal man that never liked crowds. He loved his family and just wanted to be with them. Those early days with Carl were very special and are times that I cherish.

Rico Petrocelli was also supportive and was a great example for me on how to act like a professional both on and off the field. He also would take me to chapel and that's when my relationship with God started.

Doug Griffin was another teammate I instantly became tight with because we lived in the same neighborhood and would drive to the ballpark together. Doug was also close with Carl and loved to fish, so we had those things in common, as well.

And then there was Bill "Spaceman" Lee, a media darling, who plugged me right away with the press. After I came up, he told Clif Keane, a longtime sportswriter for the *Boston Globe* and later a talk radio host on the *Clif-and-Claf Show*, that "Dwight comes out of Chatsworth, has the most beautiful swing, is graceful, and just moves so perfectly in the outfield. He could turn out to be the next DiMaggio." To which Keane, a funny character, replied, "Yeah, *Vince*." I always loved Bill, one of the game's great characters who was a fine pitcher for us. Bill still plays baseball at 77 years old for the Savannah Bananas as well as a men's league team in Vermont. He'll probably die in his uniform. He's already said that's how he wants to go. In fact, he almost did die in 2022 when he had a heart attack in the bullpen prior to a Bananas game. When the team held a meeting with him to express their concerns over what would happen if he were to die on the mound, he told them, "Just drag me to the back of the mound, take the small tarp that goes over it, throw it over me, and take care of me after the game!" And that's Bill in a nutshell. He truly loves the game and has a great sense of humor.

So I had some great relationships with some of my teammates even early on. It really wasn't like how the negative Boston media famously portrayed our club as "25 players, 25 cabs." There was unity among us.

We played well down the stretch and, after a four-game winning streak from September 27 through 30, found ourselves with a 1½-game lead with just four games left in the season. But then a 2–1 loss to the Orioles cut our lead to a half game over the Tigers as we began a three-game, season-ending series against them in Detroit. We needed to take two out of three games to clinch the division crown.

A football game had been played in the rain at Tiger Stadium the day before we arrived, and the field was an absolute mess.

As it turned out, we fell victim to the adverse conditions early in the first game. Trailing 1–0 in the top of the third with one out and Tommy Harper on third and Luis Aparicio on first, Yaz drove one into the right center field gap between Mickey Stanley and Al Kaline that looked to be a two-run triple. Harper scored, but as Aparicio was rounding third, he slipped on the wet grass. Luis got up off the ground and scampered back to third, but Yaz was already there. Carl attempted to race back to second but was tagged out. Because Aparicio slipped on the wet surface, instead of taking a 2–1 lead with one out and a man on third, it was tied at one apiece with two out with Aparicio on third. Reggie Smith, the next hitter, struck out to end the inning. What could have been a game-breaking rally was squandered, in part, due to the field conditions.

In the sixth inning, the Tigers led 3–1 with runners on first and third and two outs when Stanley hit a fly ball out to me that, at first, I lost in the lights. Once I picked up the flight of the ball again, it was behind me. Moving back, I slipped and fell as my feet went out from under me, yet I managed to catch the ball flat on my butt with my legs out in front of me to keep the game close. To this day, I still don't know how I was able to catch it. The conditions were terrible, but as players, what could we say? There was nothing we could do about it. We lost the game 4–1 to drop a half game behind the Tigers with two to play.

After losing the next game 3–1, we were eliminated. We would win the final game of the season, but it didn't matter because, due to an early season strike, we played one fewer game than the Tigers, so they won the division by half a game.

To this day, Lee blames politics for the Red Sox not winning the division. Despite going 9–2 in 1971, Kasko didn't start him in a single game in '72. Lee wore a Rolling Stones T-shirt in spring training that read LICK DICK IN '72. Kasko, who supported

President Nixon, only used Lee out of the bullpen, presumably as a form of punishment. The next season, when the Red Sox staff suffered numerous injuries, Lee was made a starter and won 17 games. I wasn't aware of the dissension between the two—I was just happy to be there—but it's safe to say had Lee started some games for us in '72, the outcome would have been better for us.

Despite the heartbreaking conclusion to the '72 campaign, there were still the usual hijinks that went on in the clubhouse. With the club already eliminated prior to the season finale, most of our starters weren't playing that day—including Aparicio. Luis wore these beautiful thousand-dollar suits back then and, after packing his bags at his locker, got dressed for his trip home to Caracas. What he soon came to realize was that Yaz, who also wasn't playing that day, had cut Luis' suit pants off above the knees, turned them inside out, and used white tape from the trainer's room to reattach the pant legs. When Luis put his pants on, the lower legs portion came off. Aparicio was furious and wanted to kill Yaz. But that was Carl—he may have been a quiet leader but he was still a prankster with a powerful clubhouse presence. He wanted to give Aparicio something to remember him by over the winter. Luis had to go through customs in Miami and on to Caracas dressed in a suit with short pants. On his way out, Aparicio kept yelling at Carl, "I'm going to get you back next year!"

Soon after the season ended, against my better judgment, I agreed to play winter ball in Venezuela. I had already played a back-breaking total of 212 games over the previous 12 months between the Instructional League, Louisville, and the Red Sox. I desperately needed some time off, Susan was pregnant with Timothy, and I just didn't want to go.

But the Red Sox sent me there to play for Luis Aparicio's Lara team because they wanted me to face good pitchers like Pete Broberg of the Texas Rangers and Roric Harrison, who had just been traded from Baltimore to Atlanta in the big Earl Williams trade. Harrison was really tough and had a good hard slider and fastball. During my time up with Boston at the end of the '72 season, I didn't see much of a difference in velocity of speed between pitchers in Triple-A and the major leagues, but the major league hurlers had better curveballs and sliders and they almost always hit their spots. So, in the sense of getting more experience hitting big league pitching, winter ball, on the surface, seemed like a good idea to the Red Sox as part of my development. Plus, Aparicio said to me, "I'm going to take care of you, we'll be good. You can get jewelry down there. Anything you ever need, I can get it for you." But when I got down to Venezuela, Luis was nowhere to be found. It turned out he really wasn't too involved with the team. When he managed, he would show up right at game time. And at times, he could really go off the rails. He had a team meeting one time and told all the USA guys to leave the clubhouse so he could address the local players privately. Out of the back of his pants, he pulled out a pistol and started threatening them with it if they didn't play better! The USA guys weren't supposed to see that, but we saw some of it and heard more about it later. As much as Aparicio was revered in the United States, and rightfully so as a great player, he was different down there.

After about half the winter league season, Luis and I got into an argument that nearly resulted in me hooking him. The thing that really touched things off with him was all the travel we had to do. We used to take these long bus trips to Caracas. You'd ride over these mountain roads on cliffs and every few miles you'd see a cross where some bus or car had gone over the edge. After a while, those bus trips started to really bother me. After a while, whenever we had a trip to Caracas, I'd fly there and meet the club. The next thing I knew, Luis started fining me for missing the team buses. I finally had enough of it, told him so, and informed him I was going back home for the rest of the winter.

But leaving Venezuela wasn't easy. When I left the team, Lara officials stopped communicating with me. So when I arrived in Caracas to catch a flight home, customs officials wouldn't let me out of Venezuela without the tax papers the team was supposed to provide me with. I actually spent 24 hours on the streets of Caracas, not knowing what to do. Finally, I got so frustrated that I called Red Sox vice president of player personnel Haywood Sullivan and told him I was stuck down there. That was a trying time for me, and Luis was largely responsible for Lara not giving me my tax papers. Ultimately, Sullivan contacted Willie Paflin, a Red Sox scout in Venezuela, who would get my tax papers and meet me at the airport so I could fly back to California.

It was great to be back home with Susan for Christmas, get some rest, and reflect on what was a whirlwind 1972. Best of all, I proved to myself that I could be called up from Triple-A and be tossed right into the thick of a tight pennant race and come through with some clutch hits and play strong defense at the big-league level.

The future was looking bright.

CHAPTER 5

TEDDY BALLGAME

TED WILLIAMS WAS UNQUESTIONABLY one of the greatest Americans of the 20th Century. First and foremost, he put his life on the line defending our country. Here was a guy who fought three years in the United States Navy and Marine Corps during World War II and another two years as a Marine combat aviator in the Korean War. It's been reported that on one mission over North Korea, his jet was so full of bullet holes that it was a miracle he kept it up in the air and then landed safely over the border into South Korea. John Wayne portrayed guys like Ted on the silver screen. For this, I had total respect for Ted—he was a very special individual.

He is also considered one of the greatest—if not *the greatest*—hitters of all-time. The list of accomplishments for the Hall of Famer on the baseball field is remarkably long. Ted was a 19-time All-Star, a two-time American League Most Valuable Player, a six-time AL batting champion, a two-time Triple Crown winner, and is the last player to hit over .400 in a season. Had he not missed five years serving in the military during the prime of his career, he very well may have broken Babe Ruth's then-record of 714 lifetime home runs.

Ted was like a mythical figure and the prospect of meeting him and talking hitting at my first Red Sox spring training was thrilling to me and one I looked forward to with great anticipation.

Alas, it would turn out to be disastrous and a source of great embarrassment.

Back then, the Red Sox had far fewer players who participated in spring training than do today. In 1973, Boston had a 40-man roster and a few invitees, and we were all on the same field during workouts. They had four mounds on the side for the pitchers with the position players on the diamond and in the outfield. One day early in spring training, I was in right field and I saw Ted Williams, who was working for the club as a special batting instructor after resigning a year earlier from a managerial post with the Texas Rangers. He was 50 feet or so behind second base and was watching batting practice. He had his arm crossed with a fungo bat hanging under his left elbow, gripping it with his right hand. As line drives were hit toward him, he leaned his head one way or the other way, lifted his right or left leg, or turned sideways, depending on the flight and direction of the batted balls, to avoid contact with them. This went on for 15 minutes when I thought, *I'm going to introduce myself to Ted*. Now, this was my first spring training and I was just 20 years old, but I mustered the courage to go up to him.

"Hi Ted, I'm Dwight Evans," I said. Ted was known for being very boisterous and his voice really carried. "*I know who you are!*" he shouted, without making any eye contact. "*I know who you are!*" Despite how uncomfortable I felt, for the next two minutes, I continued to try to talk to him—even as he still wouldn't look at me and gave me nothing but one-word answers to my questions. When I shyly and politely asked him, "What were you thinking in situations like 2-and-0 and 3-and-1?" he went *ballistic!* I swore at that time too, but he used adjectives I had never even heard of before—actually *inventing* swear words—leaving me to wonder where he came up with such stuff.

"How in the f—k can you ask me a question like that?!" he bellowed. "You're in a [insert invented swear word here] major league camp and you ask me that question?!" He went on and on with the verbiage very loudly for what felt like an eternity, then threw his fungo bat about 50 feet in the air like a baton, not knowing if it was going to come down on him or me. If I had a shovel, I would have dug myself out of there. To make matters even worse, if that's even possible, I was looking over his shoulder and, besides my teammates, I noticed quite a few fans who came to watch BP who were now watching Ted air me out. Everything came to a grinding halt, batting practice stopped, and *everybody* had their eyes on us. The ballpark was quiet except for the sound of Ted's booming voice really giving it to me. It was my worst nightmare.

Still, I tried to take the high road and did the only thing I thought appropriate under the circumstances. I simply tapped him on the shoulder and said, "Ted, it must be a bad day. I'll talk to you some other time." Then I just walked away from him. The show was over, batting practice resumed, and everything got back to normal. I walked out to right field just devastated. I didn't talk to Ted for four years after that. I just didn't have any time for him. He really was a tremendous athlete, a hero in World War II and the Korean War, and was just on another level for me as far as respect goes, but that day he lost everything I had for him.

Four years later, again during spring training, he had a bunch of us out to hit. He had the cage set up after a game, a guy throwing BP, and a few others shagging fly balls. "You've got to hit with your g—damn hips!" he yelled at us like we couldn't hear him. After about 10 minutes of us hitting pop-ups in the cage and high one-hoppers to the third baseman, he started screaming at us, walked away, and left us all there—session over. Ted simply couldn't teach hitting. Sometimes you have geniuses in other professions like in science who are just so intelligent in their field but can't teach what they know. That was Ted.

Worse yet, he couldn't accept people that couldn't perform the way he did, because he was so great and simply couldn't teach it. And that included some of his best friends in baseball, such as Hall of Famer Bobby Doerr. Bobby was a sweetheart of a man from Oregon. But they would sometimes go at it when Ted would start sharing his beliefs and philosophies about hitting.

Years later, Ted would give Walt Hriniak, who was a phenomenal hitting coach for the Red Sox, tremendous grief over his methods. He felt Walt was setting baseball back, robbing hitters of extra-base hits and home runs by teaching them to hit the ball up the middle. Walt also talked about swinging level and then, once you make contact, finishing up. Ted taught swinging at a 5- to 6-percent angle from level-to-up. Additionally, Walt was all about being disciplined with your head, and I'll go to my grave totally believing that. If your head is not down (for example, if you're right-handed, and already looking at third base) in that moment of truth when the bat meets the ball, you're in trouble. You might still get a hit, but you won't know how you got it. Walt was big on these points, and, to this day, I talk about them with Red Sox hitters. But Ted just didn't understand what Walt was teaching and took issue with several Red Sox players, including myself, who became Hriniak-hitting disciples.

Before one spring training game in 1982, Ted came into our Winter Haven clubhouse with his usual entourage of five or six people who all called him "Teddy Ballgame." Once you came around the wall into the clubhouse, my locker was on the right. Looking right at me, he bellowed out, "I'll be g—damned if I teach anybody to swing down on the ball." Of course, his little cronies start saying things like, *That a boy, Teddy Ballgame, you tell him!* and that kind of thing. But it was kind of funny at the same time.

I let this go on for a while before finally saying to him, "Ted, you know I don't know anything about aerodynamics, and I didn't go to college." Williams cut me off and snapped, "I figured that!" Ignoring his comeback, I continued, "While not knowing anything about aerodynamics, Ted, I do know something about going from point A to point B." I then demonstrated this by drawing a straight line on a piece of paper and then, to show his philosophy, a line with a little loop to it. "I know one thing, Ted," I continued. "If I go from Point A to Point B in a straight line, wouldn't that be quicker than with a loop in it?" Ted knew where I was going with this, and I thought I had him. But he just got agitated and started shouting, "Ahhh! You just don't know!" And he walked away while one of his cronies said, "Way to go, Teddy Ballgame!" It was one of those times I thought, *I got him on that one.*

But here's the crazy thing. Over the years, he came to like and respect me. He just had a gruff way of showing it. In 1994, he opened the Ted Williams Museum and Hitters Hall of Fame in Hernando, Florida. In 2002, the last year of his life, he inducted me into it in a class that included Cal Ripken Jr. and Enos "Country" Slaughter. That kind of recognition made me feel good because everybody talks about me as being a great defensive player with a strong arm, but I always come back to them with, "I could hit, too."

After the induction ceremony, I went to Ted's home. He had recently had heart surgery and his voice was weak. Now confined to a wheelchair, he wheeled over to me and said softly, "You should have been a better hitter than you were." I took it as a compliment and, coming from Ted, it meant a lot to me, because he threw out compliments like manhole covers. Even though he really thought I should have been better, he had just inducted me into his Hall of Fame, an honor he didn't extend to a lot of other guys who were in the Baseball Hall of Fame.

I came around to thinking Ted was a neat guy, especially after doing some research on the challenges he had growing up. He didn't have a father around and his mother worked for the Salvation Army in San Diego, yet he turned out to be a true American hero.

After the humiliation of my Ted Williams encounter, I had to quickly let it go. Even though I was MVP of the International League and then came up and did a nice job down the pennant stretch for the Red Sox the year before, I had a job to fight for that spring. There were no guarantees, especially after we signed future Hall of Famer Orlando Cepeda that winter. But after the signing, Kasko said that if Cepeda couldn't play regularly at first base, then Yaz would be moved there from left field, opening a spot in the outfield. It was quickly determined that Cepeda would be used as our first designated hitter and that Yaz would, in fact, play primarily at first. It was also decided that Tommy Harper would be the regular left fielder with Reggie Smith moving to center. This meant that right field—and the last roster spot—was up for grabs between Cecil Cooper, a great ballplayer who would go on to have a wonderful career, and me. Our competition went on all spring training long and came down to the last exhibition game. Kasko called us both into his office and said, "It's between you guys. It's a tough decision, but we can only take one of you." Our fate would literally come down to our last at-bats of that final game. I doubled down the left field line and Cooper popped out. I went north with the club to Boston; Cooper went to Triple-A. It was that close.

One of the perks of making the club was getting to change my uniform number from the No. 40 they assigned to me to my favorite—No. 24. Twenty-four was my favorite because that's the number my idol, Willie Mays, wore. When I was 10 years old and growing up in LA, when I would see the Dodgers play the Giants, Mays always struck me as a player I could emulate and model myself after. I always tried to make basket catches like he did in little league. To me, he was the greatest player of all time. He could hit, run, throw, and his instincts were off the charts. He didn't really need a coach for running the bases. His helmet would fly off and he knew exactly where he was and what he could and couldn't do. He could also steal bases but not worry about breaking records—he would only steal in situations that called for it.

Mays' last year in baseball was in 1973 with the Mets. That spring training, we went over to play the Mets at Al Lang Stadium in St. Petersburg. During batting practice, Mays was in right field playing catch and warming up. I looked over and badly wanted to introduce myself to him. I was shy, but I finally got up enough nerve to start walking in his direction. But at that very moment, batting practice ended, and he ran off the field—an opportunity lost.

However, later in life, when I was a coach with Colorado, we were in San Francisco and Mays walked through the coaches' room. Even after my 20-year playing career, I looked at him and was still somewhat speechless. He was just so special in my book. But I did manage to make some small talk with him this time. A smile still comes across my face just thinking about the memories of watching him play.

As the Red Sox went north for our '73 season opener, I hoped that some of Mays' magical No. 24 would rub off on me.

CHAPTER 6

ONE TRYING SEASON

"THIS IS YOUR JOB," Eddie Kasko told me in right field before an early season game in 1973. "No matter what, you're going to be out here, so you don't have to worry." Five games later, as my hitting slump continued, he started platooning me. So, after his vote of confidence, I had a nice little journey as the regular right fielder for about a week.

As a right-handed hitter, I was encouraged by the club to adapt my hitting style to take advantage of the 37-foot-tall Green Monster, which appeared so close from home plate. But that made me a lousy hitter early in the season because my power was from right-center to left-center. But now, because of the Monster, they wanted me to pull the ball. Fenway can change you if you don't receive the proper instruction and without coaches telling you to stay with your strengths as a hitter. When I came up, we didn't have any defined hitting coaches, and nobody really worked with you. Eddie Popowski, who I loved, would shout, "Grab a piece of cheese and wrap it around the pole!" What that meant in baseball terminology was to get a fastball and pull it. I would never say that to a young player today. About 75 percent of pitches are designed to be middle-away. So, if you're going to be a pull-hitter, you're looking for 25 percent of the pitches that will be middle-in.

But most pitchers don't like pitching in. Usually if it's in, it's *way in* and a ball, and it's used to set up pitches to the outside part of the plate. But as a kid, I didn't know any of this and just did what I was told.

I was still only 21 and probably could have used a little more seasoning. The biggest jump that I had as a professional may have been moving from Single-A straight to Triple-A, though it would take me much of the first half of the '73 season to fully adjust to big league pitching. But when I did, I showed what I could do. In one weekend that August in Texas, I hit two doubles, two home runs—including a 450-foot blast off Steve Dunning that, at the time, was the second longest in Arlington Stadium history—and scored six runs. But in the top of the seventh of the final game of the series, I was seriously beaned by Texas pitcher Mike Paul. I lost sight of the pitched ball in Paul's uniform and, as I turned my head, it hit me right behind my left ear and knocked me out for 20 seconds. I had to come out of the game and was sent to the hospital where I spent the night. My head hurt really bad. They hadn't yet identified the symptoms of a concussion in baseball— nor did they know how to treat it.

The team flew to Anaheim, the next stop on our road trip, without me, and after I rejoined the team after missing the next game, Kasko came up to me to ask how I was feeling. I said, "Lightheaded, but I'm okay." He then asked if I could play. Even though I probably should have said I shouldn't, there was no way I was going to say no back then.

We would face Nolan Ryan that evening in a game starting at 6:05 PM. Ryan always pitched at twilight whenever possible, taking full advantage of when the shadows only cover the infield. The stadium lights would be on, but all you could see was a sil-houette of Ryan. You couldn't really pick up his features with the outfield sun shining brightly behind him, a very unsettling feeling for hitters when facing the man they called "the Ryan Express" because of how hard he threw. As I came up to bat for the first time that game, the Angels' catcher, Jeff Torborg, said, "Dewey, how are you feeling?" I said, "Jeff, I'm doing okay. Thanks for asking. I'm just lightheaded." I got in the batter's box, Ryan wound up and delivered his first pitch—and I never saw it. Thank God I never saw it, because if I had, it may have killed me. Ryan threw the pitch behind my head. If a pitcher is trying to hit you in the head, that's exactly where he throws it, because your first natural instinct is to move back to avoid it.

I stepped out of the box and glared at Ryan, and then I looked down at Torborg. My mind was telling me to wrap Torborg over the head with my bat and charge the mound, but they had a guy named Mike Epstein at first base who was about 6'4" and 240 pounds and another guy at third base, Bob Oliver, who was 6'3" and 245 pounds. I quickly evaluated the situation with my head hurting like it was and thought, *I'm going to be right back in the hospital if I charge that mound.* So I stayed in the batter's box.

Not that Ryan would care, but I lost all respect for him after that. He had a great career and he probably either wouldn't remember the incident today or would say he didn't try to throw at me, but he had pretty good control. I nearly took the ultimate revenge later in the at-bat when I hit a long fly ball to right center field that Leroy Stanton caught high against the wall—just missing a home run. It kind of proved that throwing at my head was not going to intimidate me. And I would prove that again by taking him deep a couple of seasons later at Fenway. I would never allow Ryan to get inside my head. Still, that purposeful pitch he threw behind my head right after my serious beaning was a tough moment.

Although my hitting had been inconsistent that season, my defense, which I took a lot of pride in, was solid, and I committed just one error in 183 chances. I had a good arm and a quick release. I never had any fears in the outfield and always wanted the ball hit to me.

I also quickly adapted to the nuances of Fenway's challenging right field, which I always believed was the most difficult to navigate in baseball. People have said to me things like, *Well, you play at Fenway, so of course you think it's the hardest.* But it really is.

First, it's one of the biggest right fields in all of baseball. It goes from Pesky's Pole, where it's only 302 feet, almost directly to 380 in straight-away right field. Second, there's really no foul territory. That's because after first base where the grounds crew area comes into play, it ends. So, if a ball lands anywhere out there, it's fair. Third, the angles are unlike anywhere else. You would see right fielders from other teams go out there for three or four games a couple of times a year and it would just screw them up. When I was in right and faced home plate, the side to my left was a whole different animal than when a ball was hit to the right of me. If it were hit hard and hooking past first base, it usually kicked off the area by the grounds crew and you could hold the runner to a single. But if it went straight past the grounds crew area and up the line, you had to really bust it and run directly at Pesky's Pole to cut it off and hold the runner to a double, because if it got by you and rolled around the corner, it could end up being a triple or an inside-the-park home run. And fourth, dealing with the sun was brutal. Back then, the stadium was low and hadn't been built up like it is today. The low grandstand made the sun nasty to contend with, and I'm lucky I don't have issues with my eyes now because of all the years I spent looking up at it during day games. I likely had the darkest flip-down glasses in baseball to protect them. The sun also created shadows in the infield, making it almost impossible to tell if a ball was hit off the end of the bat or hit solidly—affecting your jump on the ball.

I also had to adjust to the hitters around the league. The one that made me the most uneasy in right field was Tony Oliva, one of the great left-handed hitters of his generation. Usually, when a ball is hit directly at you in right, you automatically turn toward the line because the ball is going to hook. With Oliva, sometimes the ball would hook, but other times it would go the other way because he kind of inside-outed it that way. He was like Vladimir Guerrero, a right-handed hitter, who would take a ball low and in and hit it out to right center; or take a ball away and pull it to left field. He's the kind of guy that if you're a hitting coach you leave alone and don't say anything to him. Oliva was the same way. As a right fielder, you could usually kind of cheat if you knew what pitch was coming, but with Oliva, you couldn't. Another guy who would give me fits was Graig Nettles. Nettles would hit Björn Borg–like serves to right field. He swung up on the ball and he'd hit a line drive that looked like it was going out of the ballpark, so your first step would be to turn back; but suddenly, it would take this big spin and drop in front of you. So, Oliva and Nettles made me very uncomfortable in the outfield.

Despite all the adjustments and the ebbs and flows of the '73 season, nothing could prepare Susan and I for the news we received late that August. Timothy was just six months old when his left eyelid started getting puffy. At first, it was believed to be a closed tear duct, a condition affecting approximately 20 percent of newborns where tears can't drain normally, though it usually resolves on its own within six months. But we soon found out from Dr. Charles Byer at Massachusetts Eye and Ear Hospital in Boston that was not the case. Dr. Byer would diagnose Timothy's condition as Neurofibromatosis (NF), a genetic disorder that produces benign but painful soft tumors on the nerves. When those tumors are hit, it is very painful. It's like going to the dentist's office and they blow air into a filling, irritating the nerves.

The manifestation of NF leads to learning disabilities—one of the milder parts of it—as well as tumor deformity, before advancing to cancer. It's a life-threatening disease that, over time, the patient succumbs to.

It's hard when you're an athlete and something's not right with your child. It's difficult on your wife, too. We didn't know how his malady came about and why. We kept asking ourselves, *Why is this happening to us?* and *Why is it happening to Timothy?* It would be the beginning of a very tough life for him—and a trying time for our young family.

The club finished the '73 campaign in second place, eight games behind the Orioles in the AL East. For me personally, a poor year at the plate without question cost me playing time. The Red Sox, a contender all season long, had outfield depth and, because of that, whenever I slumped at the plate, it meant time on the bench. Had I played for a non-contender, I would have played more and settled into my big-league rookie year. But I wouldn't have traded playing for the Red Sox for anything. I was more about wanting to win than getting caught up with my own accomplishments. It was the example that was instilled in me that season by Yaz, Petrocelli, Harper, Tiant, and Reggie Smith. It was all about winning in Boston. There's no better time to be playing than when you've got a chance to get into a World Series. And I knew, with the club we had, we would get that chance sooner rather than later.

CHAPTER 7

OUR TIME HAD COME

THE BOSTON WRITERS and talk shows had a field day following the 1974 season, labeling us "choke artists." With less than six weeks left in the campaign, we squandered a seven-game lead to finish in third place, seven games out. But we didn't feel like choke artists at all. The division-winning Orioles finished the season on a torrid pace, winning 28 of their final 34 games. And although we were just 13–21 over that same period, the ballgames we lost were generally close and well played.

We also suffered through some significant injuries, most notably the one to Carlton Fisk that ended his season on June 28. We were in Cleveland and, with the game tied at 1–1 in the bottom of the ninth and Leron Lee on first, George Hendrick doubled to left field. With Lee charging home, the relay throw from the outfield into shortstop Mario Guerrero was a good one, but Mario double-pumped, and his throw home was late enough for Fisk, who was blocking the plate, to get bowled over—badly damaging his knee as a result. I went up to the trainer's room to check on Carlton after the game to see just how severe the injury was. The doctor that was examining him moved his knee laterally both ways. It was totally blown out, requiring major knee surgery.

Despite all of this, as we entered the '75 season, the press was brutal. They wrote us off. We were like the Rodney Dangerfield of baseball—no respect. The Yankees, who finished just two games out in '74, had added Cy Young Award winner Catfish Hunter in free agency and traded for five-tool outfielder Bobby Bonds, making them the media's favorite to win the American League East. The Orioles appeared to improve themselves further with the additions of sluggers Lee May and Ken Singleton, and pitcher Mike Torrez, and were largely picked to finish in second place. And the Milwaukee Brewers, who had a losing record in '74 and had only added an aging Hank Aaron during the off-season, were inexplicably slated to finish in third. Somehow, we were predicted to be a fourth-place team by the so-called experts. The critics claimed that we hadn't done anything in the off-season to improve ourselves.

Hadn't the writers seen the talent we had returning? I thought.

We would have "the Gold Dust Twins," outfielders Fred Lynn and Jim Rice—both of whom played brilliantly when called up late in the '74 season—for an entire season. They had jumped right in and took over where they left off in Triple-A to put big numbers on the board. It was inexplicable why they weren't played more. When Lynn came up in September, he just sat on the bench for the first two weeks, then went out and hit .419 in 15 games. Jimmy had been called up in mid-August, appeared in roughly only half the games, and was a real run-producer when he had the opportunity. While we struggled mightily as a team to score runs the last six weeks of the season, Johnson wasn't using the Gold Dust Twins nearly as much as he could have, which was strange, especially in Freddie's case, because Lynn played for Johnson in the Triple-A World Series, so Darrell knew what Lynn could do. I suppose it was possible that Johnson was apprehensive about putting rookies into the heat of a pennant race. But with Lynn and Rice on the opening day roster in '75, it would instantly change the dynamic of our ball club tremendously.

We were also due to get Fisk back sometime in the first half of the season, and had Yaz, Petrocelli, and Burleson coming off strong seasons. Tiant and Lee were still in their prime and were the anchors of the pitching staff. So I didn't understand the negativity and lack of optimism coming from the press. To me it didn't matter, because we believed in ourselves.

I put it together offensively, as well, the previous season, hitting .281 and driving in 70 runs due, in part, to playing more and having a great lineup around me. And in right field, I went 191 games without an error in 1973–74, the sixth-best streak in American League history, while beginning to get a reputation as a guy you couldn't run on.

Prior to the '74 season, Darrell Johnson took over as the Sox manager, and I'm certain that had a lot to do with my improvement. Darrell was my manager at Triple-A when I was MVP, so he knew me and had confidence in me—and vice versa. We had a great relationship, and I loved the guy. It wasn't lost on me what he told the Boston scribes late in the '74 season, "Dwight is already the best defensive right fielder in the league. And he's shown us that he has the ability at the plate to develop into a consistent offensive threat." I don't know how my teammates felt about him, but when you have a manager like that in your corner, it makes a tremendous difference.

Don Zimmer, then our third base coach, was just as encouraging, telling reporters, "Evans is going to be a solid .300 hitter in a year or so. There are certain types of pitchers who give him trouble right now, but Dewey is going to overcome that in time."

Soon thereafter, Boston writer Bill Leston wrote a feature story about how I would become a worthy successor to Ted Williams and Yaz. I probably had Darrell and Zim to thank for some of that.

But I never sought fame. I just wanted to put it all together—*my whole game*—and was gaining confidence day-by-day that I would get there. It was a goal I worked tirelessly to accomplish.

So, in my own mind, as nice as Leston's article was, I didn't need to be exonerated in the newspaper. When you're playing, and your emotions are so fragile, to read something about yourself—negative or even positive—in the sports section or listening to the talk shows can be counterproductive. After all, I already knew what I did in the last game. I didn't have to relive it. It was around this time that Susan would hand me the newspaper *without* the sports section in it.

But with Boston being the sixth largest media market in the country, it wasn't always easy to block it all out. Zimmer once told me he didn't listen to sports shows and then, shortly thereafter, he dove right into a sports talk guy for something he said earlier that day on the air. I said to him, "Hey Zim, I thought you weren't listening to those guys!"

To become a better ballplayer, I needed to have a short memory. It was the same during a game. If I hit a home run my first time up, I wasn't going to live off that my second time to the plate. As a hitter, it's better to bring it down to one at-bat at a time and, if you can, the optimum scenario is one *pitch* at a time. Putting all your concentration and energy into each pitch is the ultimate in baseball. I knew some guys who knew exactly what their batting average was if they went 2-for-3 or 3-for-4—right down to the decimal point. I couldn't do that. It would put too much pressure on me.

———————

Away from the ballpark at the start of the '75 season, life was difficult and complicated. Timothy had just had his first NF-related surgery at two years old and had to wear a patch over his left eye that spring. Susan was pregnant with Kirstin, and we were deeply concerned that if Timothy had NF, what issues would our newborn daughter have? But we didn't have a way of checking back then on whether a child would be born with NF.

One of my challenges then as a professional ballplayer was to try my best to compartmentalize my family life and my baseball life. Prior to the '75 season, I lacked some of the confidence in my everyday life a player needs to reach their full potential. Aside from not having an ego, I had a son who was sick, which brought me down to earth more than anything. It's hard to be confident when deeply upsetting things are going on in your life. I was confused and didn't really know what was going on. I kind of wish I had some therapy to go to or something that could have helped me out. I didn't know God then, but I was blaming Him for everything that was happening to Timothy. I was *mad* at somebody I didn't even know.

Despite the challenges, I was determined to get off to a great start for the '75 campaign—and I did. Through one-third of the season, I was among the Red Sox leaders in runs, hits, doubles, triples, RBIs, and walks. And in a key situation in a game against the Oakland A's that May in Fenway Park, I held Reggie Jackson at third base on a fly ball hit to medium right field—proving to opponents that they challenge my arm at their own risk.

We really came together as a team that May. The club was invigorated by our young players with a hard-nosed style of play that was resonating with the Boston fans. You had Lynn diving and leaping for balls all over the outfield and Burleson going deep into the hole at short to make plays. It was extra-special because of what happened the year before. We showed them that we had some chutzpah and that we weren't going to cave in this time.

I connected with Lynn in center field right away. We were like one. We listened to each other, let one another know where we were playing, and communicated constantly—even using hand signals when the crowd got loud. I played with some great centerfielders, but Freddie was the best of them all. I may have gone on to win eight Gold Gloves, but I always gave credit to the guy next to me because I wouldn't have won those awards if I didn't have a great centerfielder out there with me. What was nice was when Freddie won four Gold Gloves when he played alongside me and when I won three of mine while sharing the outfield with him.

Over in left field, Yaz and Rice were splitting time, giving us one of the finest defensive outfields in baseball—a defense that was often overshadowed because of how good our offense was.

After a doubleheader split in Kansas City on June 13, we were tied with the Yankees for first. The next day, we made a trade with the California Angels for Denny Doyle which, at the time, didn't seem all that significant. We already had Doug Griffin at second base and Denny had barely played that season with the Angels. But once Denny got an opportunity to play, he shined and quickly became our regular second baseman. Doyle was a fiery, sparkplug kind of player who was a great addition to the club.

Before Denny's first game starting at second base for us, he said to me, "Dewey, do you want signs?" I said, "What are you talking about?" "You want the pitches? I'll give them to you," he said. So, when we were out in the field, right before a pitch, he would flash something behind his back. Our pitchers would complain when he did that, contending that the other team could relay the signs to the opposing hitter from the bullpen. But that was ridiculous. There's no way on earth that would happen. At that point, a hitter's attention is on trying to pick up the arm slot where the ball is being thrown from. They're not looking out at the right field bullpen at a guy flashing a card saying, "It's a fastball!" The pitch would already be by him. Besides, I would constantly change the signs from game to game, inning to inning and sometimes even hitter to hitter. I always loved our pitchers, but I just never understood their logic sometimes. Anyway, because I knew what pitch was coming, I could play the outfield like an infielder. Infielders always knew exactly what pitch was coming and could cheat one way or another. If a hitter is left-handed and you're at first or second base, you cheat knowing that if it's a breaking ball, he's not going to lace it to left field—he's going to pull it. If it's a fastball, you might hold your ground depending on the hitter. But being in the outfield and knowing what was coming changed me completely and made me a better player. Denny brought that to me and when he left the club, I had all our future second basemen—Jerry Remy, Marty Barrett, and Jody Reed—do the same.

A few days later, on June 17, Rice would achieve almost mythical status for his strength during a game in Detroit. Already getting a lot of attention for being one of the league leaders in home runs, Jimmy checked his swing on a pitch and the bat *snapped* in half. I had never seen that before. *Nobody* had. It was remarkable to see. Jimmy never worked out but was just so naturally strong. He had one of the strongest body types—in his quads and his back—I've ever seen. Jimmy was farm strong. His only workouts were baseball-related, and he did what he needed to do to stay in shape that way. Shortly thereafter, Hank Aaron would say, "If anyone breaks my home run record, it will be Jim Rice."

The next night, it was Freddie's turn to make headlines when he hit three home runs, a triple, and a single and had 10 RBIs in Tiger Stadium. Two nights earlier, Mickey Lolich had snapped Lynn's 20-game hitting streak. Still upset about his hitting streak ending a couple of days later, Freddie got up early in the morning and wandered around the streets of downtown Detroit, a rookie mistake—especially back in those days. We both arrived at Tiger Stadium early at around 2:00 PM and he asked me to throw batting practice to him. Like most outfielders, I usually threw terrible BP and Freddie would get so mad at me. Outfielders are notorious for throwing lousy batting practice because we have a long arm slot that goes back behind the lower back down by our thigh and then up and over. Anyway, it might have been the only time I threw him a lot of good strikes and, as a result, he got into a good rhythm, hitting line drives while getting his frustrations about losing his hitting streak out of his system.

After his big game, I went up to him and asked, "Do you want me to throw you BP tomorrow?" He gave me a huge smile. That was one of the best days I've seen *any* player have. Lynn was now hitting .352 with 14 home runs and 50 RBI. Comparisons to Stan Musial were being drawn.

The entire nation was now paying attention to us. NBC started putting us on the *Game of the Week* regularly. We knew we were special. For as much as Lynn and Rice were capturing the imagination of the baseball world, it wasn't just about them or about Freddie's big night. It was never one specific thing that was making us the team to watch. There was a culmination of factors at play. If it wasn't Lynn or Rice having a big game at the plate, it was Yaz or Fisk or Cecil Cooper or Petrocelli or myself. If it wasn't Tiant or Lee pitching a gem, it was Rick Wise, Reggie Cleveland, or Roger Moret. If it wasn't Denny making a big play in the infield, it was the Rooster. We were a deep team without any significant flaws.

And we got better and stronger as the season went along. Aside from stealing Doyle from the Angels for a song and a dance, Carlton Fisk returned to the club for the first time since breaking his forearm thanks to a pitched ball in spring training on June 23. Then when Darrell moved Roger Moret from the bullpen into the starting rotation at the end of June, we really took off. Roger was a skinny kid who knew how good he was. His delivery where he released the ball was sneaky, which means the ball gets on you quicker than anticipated. His nickname was "the Whip" because of the speed of the fastball he fired at hitters with that long and thin left arm. His first starting assignment was on June 29th against the Yankees where he pitched a complete game—outdueling Catfish Hunter 3–2—to move the Red Sox into first place by half a game. Making Roger a starter was one of the best decisions Johnson made all year.

As July rolled around, we began drawing big, highly enthusiastic crowds at Fenway. And with all the youth we had on the club, and with Boston being such a college town, we really bonded with the students sitting in the bleachers and around the ballpark. I couldn't count how many times I heard guys tell me they were at Boston University, Boston College, MIT, Harvard, Tufts, Emerson, and the other great colleges and universities in the Back Bay vicinity. They could get into the bleachers for a buck-and-a-quarter back then or, as some of them did, watch the game for free by sitting along the billboard beyond the centerfield bleachers with their legs draped over the edge.

I came up so young and was joined by guys like Cooper, Burleson, Rice, Lynn, Juan Beníquez, and Tim Blackwell—all of us in our early twenties in '75—playing in a major city on a team that had a chance to win it all for the first time since 1967. That's why the makeup of that team resonated with more young people than usual. They were like, *Hey, that could be me out there!* We were instantly identifiable with the fan base because we were of the same generation. To this day, people not much younger than me come up to me and say they watched me play when they were in college. It was a great memory for them, going to school in Boston and watching a team like we had.

What's downplayed so much is what a great ballpark Fenway is to watch a game in. I've been to Wrigley, the only place comparable to Fenway. It's also a wonderfully historic ballpark to view a game with great fans there, as well, but there's just something about Fenway that's extra special, and it was an honor and privilege for me to play there. The Red Sox are New England, and you must remember that New England isn't just Massachusetts, but it's also Rhode Island, Connecticut, Vermont, New Hampshire and Maine—a huge swath of the Northeast. And the Red Sox fan base extends into nearby Upstate New York, Quebec, and Nova Scotia. So, Fenway was and remains a huge venue for so many millions of fans to attend a Red Sox game.

We would go 22–11 in July and put the Yankees away late that month by taking three out of four games against them at Shea Stadium—including back-to-back shutouts by Lee and Moret—to push them 10 games back. So much for the experts predicting a title for them.

When we returned home after the Yankees series on July 28, we were on NBC's *Monday Night Baseball* and would defeat the Brewers 7–6 on a walk-off single by Fisk—who went 4-for-4 with two home runs and 5 RBIs that game—in the bottom of the ninth. We now led the AL East by a season-high nine games and the Fenway Faithful in the bleachers stayed long after the game was over, chanting, "We're Number One!" repeatedly. Pennant fever was gripping New England and it felt differently than it had in '72 and '74. We still had work to do, but there was more a sense of invincibility at play with this ball club than in past seasons when we held—and ultimately lost—leads late in the season.

I really started to bond with Yaz that summer, as we both were staying at the same hotel by Logan Airport toward the end of the season. Susan was six months pregnant with Kirstin that August and had returned home to California to be with her parents, so

I was on my own. Carl was really good to me, and it especially meant a lot to me during that time. He was 12 years my senior, yet we spent a lot of time together. Carl was a staunch Catholic and had attended Notre Dame on a basketball scholarship, so we met a lot of his priest acquaintances wherever we would go. As a child, I never went to church and was never even baptized. So, it wasn't just a teammate bond with Yaz, it was a spiritual one, as well. He was the one who started taking me to church and where I found religion. Years later, he would joke with me, saying, "You've gone too far," to which I replied, "Well, Carl, you're the one that started taking me to church in the first place."

We would also visit his parents, Carl Sr. and Hattie, at their apartment in Andover. Carl Sr. was a chiseled, hardworking man of Polish decent who supported the Yastrzemskis for years on his potato farm in Southampton, Long Island, in New York. Hattie, also of Polish descent, was so precious. She was suffering from cancer at the time yet, despite her condition, still had a playful side about her. One time when I was over there for lunch, she snuck under the table and tickled my feet! I didn't know *what* it was! She could be a real prankster and gave me a hard time in a nice way.

There were many days when Carl would take Hattie to her doctor's appointments for cancer treatment, while Susan and I did what we could for our Timothy in his battle with NF. Those weren't easy times for Carl or me. So, while I had some great friendships and rapport with my other teammates, there was more substance with Carl than the others. He was like a big brother to me.

———————

On September 21, we held a 3½-game lead in the AL East with just six games to play. While we had not clinched the division title yet, we were very close and certainly were looking a little ahead to the postseason with all the talent we had. But then, just as everything was rolling along for us, the unexpected happened. We were playing a Sunday day game in Detroit when Tigers pitcher Vern Ruhle threw an inside pitch that rode way inside to Rice. Jimmy twisted his body and leaned back as he attempted to get out of the way of the ball but was hit squarely on his left hand—fracturing it badly—and was out for the season, including the playoffs and World Series.

Losing Rice was a big blow to us. You look at the year Jimmy had and, if it weren't for Lynn, he would have likely been the one to win both the Rookie of the Year and MVP awards. It really was like splitting hairs as far as which of the two were better in '75. It was almost unfair what happened to Jimmy, which took him out of the running for those two awards and, most importantly, forced one of our outstanding young players to sit out and watch the playoffs and World Series. I will always think about what could have been had Rice been in our lineup in the postseason. It very well may have changed the course of baseball history.

Still, we were above the situation, not below it. We weren't going to let Rice's injury bring us down. There was no quit in us. If that had happened to any one of us, we would have handled it the same way. We had such a deep team and had Cecil Cooper, Bernie Carbo, and Juan Beníquez ready to step it up, knowing what was required. And we had Yaz, still an outstanding outfielder, who could move from first base back out to left field.

We would come back and defeat the Tigers 6–5 in the game in which we lost Rice, and we would keep on winning right up until we had our ace, Luis Tiant, on the mound for us in the potential division-clincher at Fenway later that week. Luis had been practically untouchable pitching at Fenway the last month of the season. It was during that month that the chants of 'Loo-ie! Loo-ie! Loo-ie!' filled the air at home games. It was as if Luis willed us to win the division. He could flat-out pitch. He could throw hard, knew how to change speeds, and regularly kept hitters off-stride. After he was done warming up prior to his starts, I would hear that bullpen door latch open and then, suddenly, you'd have about 35,000 fans rise to their feet and give him a standing ovation as he walked to our dugout with a pitching coach. He would throw his jacket on the bench and say, "Let's go!" And that standing ovation wouldn't end until he threw his first pitch. It still gives me goosebumps thinking about how I witnessed such a spectacle.

It seemed like every time Luis pitched it was against Nolan Ryan or the other team's No. 1 guy. There was no question that Tiant was the ace of our staff. And I'm not taking anything away from guys like Bill Lee. Lee may have done some quirky things between starts that made people uncomfortable, but none of that stuff bothered me. He got his work in and once he stepped over that white line to go to the mound, *nobody* was more serious about the game than him.

True to his stature as a big-game pitcher, Luis didn't disappoint in the September 26 division clincher, going the distance and hurling a four-hit shutout over the Indians. With the tough divisional losses of '72 and '74, we would have been forgiven if we thought about how extra sweet this title was. But as a team, we learned not to look back and to live in the moment. We were all about what was next and what we could still accomplish. It's true that we won the AL East by 4½ games, and it was a great time in our lives as a team, but we knew what lay ahead—a date with the Oakland A's, winners of the last three World Series.

We were no longer the "choke artists" the Boston media portrayed us as and had proven all those preseason prognosticators wrong. The Boston Red Sox were back in the postseason and Fenway Park, in all its glory, would host the first two games of the American League Championship Series the next week. I could hardly wait for the series to begin.

Naturally, the press and everyone was saying we didn't belong in the same ballpark as the mighty Oakland A's. And we knew the A's were tough. How could a team gunning for its fourth straight world championship not be? Despite losing Catfish, they still had good pitching, played sound defense, and were an excellent clutch-hitting team. They still had the nucleus of their early '70s dynasty—a lineup that included Reggie Jackson, Joe Rudi, Sal Bando, Gene Tenace, and Billy North; starting pitchers Vida Blue and Ken Holtzman; and the best reliever in the game in Rollie Fingers.

But we were confident going into the ALCS. During the regular season, we split our 12 games with the A's and had a good read on their pitchers—averaging nearly six runs a game against them. Our pitching was a little bit underrated, probably because our offense and defense got most of the headlines. I figured if we could keep the ball in the ballpark against those guys, we had a heck of a shot to beat them. We knew we were good and could compete against anybody.

As it turned out, we just smoked them, sweeping Oakland in three straight games. Everybody was hitting the A's quality pitching and they couldn't get us out in key situations. We had four of our regulars—Burleson, Cooper, Fisk, and Yaz—all hit .400 or higher for the series, and our pitchers were stellar with a 1.67 ERA.

But it was Tiant's performance that really stood out. He continued to dominate as he had all month long, going the distance in Game 1 without yielding an earned run. What made it even sweeter for Luis was having his father, Luis "Lefty" Tiant Sr., a former Negro Leagues star pitcher, and his mother, Isabel, in the stands watching him perform. Prior to that August, Luis hadn't seen Isabel for eight years and Lefty for 15 due to the severing of U.S.–Cuban diplomatic relations in 1961. It didn't hurt that Cuban ruler Fidel Castro was a huge baseball fan, working out a deal with Senator George McGovern to arrange the Tiant couple's visit to Boston to spend time with their only son. Lefty and Isabel soaked in Luis' success as El Tiante delivered some of the best pitching of his career. It would be the feel-good story of the postseason.

And now, with a trip to the World Series against the Big Red Machine, we would try to write our own bit of history and bring home the first Red Sox title since 1918.

CHAPTER 8

THE GREATEST WORLD SERIES

WHEN THE 1975 FALL CLASSIC BEGAN, there was no way of knowing that it would turn out to be *the* all-time Fall Classic. For sustained drama, with its back-and-forth lead changes, fabled home runs, spectacular defensive plays, two extra-inning contests, and five of the seven games being decided by a single run, it would be the World Series by which all others would be measured by—the da Vinci of October baseball.

Just like our series against the Oakland A's, we weren't supposed to compete with the legendary Cincinnati Reds—another David versus Goliath scenario. Most observers wondered, *Will the Reds beat them in four games or five?* After all, the '75 Reds were positively stacked with one of the greatest lineups in baseball history. They had the eventual all-time hits leader in Pete Rose leading off, followed by three future Hall of Famers in Joe Morgan, Johnny Bench, and Tony Pérez. And rounding out their starting eight were George Foster—possibly their most dangerous hitter at the time—perennial All-Star shortstop Dave Concepción, the superb Ken Griffey, and all-around threat Cesar Geronimo. The Reds also had a deep starting pitching staff; six pitchers had double figures in wins, led by their ace Don Gullett. Their bullpen, led by closer Rawly Eastwick, was just as impressive, boasting four relievers with sub-3.00 ERAs. The Reds could do it all—run, hit, hit for power, pitch, and play stellar defense. Despite all the preparation and studying every report we could get on the Reds, we knew we faced a tremendous challenge against the Big Red Machine. But we also knew we were a hot ball club that finished up the regular season strong and then pummeled the A's in every facet of the game in the ALCS.

It was also the last "pure" World Series. The free agency system would arrive that off-season and change the landscape and dynamics of Major League baseball forever. We had 19 home-grown players on our '75 World Series team, with the others coming to us by trade. You couldn't go out and improve your team by signing great players yet.

The first two games of the World Series would be played at Fenway—both *day games*—something you would never see happen today. As a kid, I never missed a World Series game, as night games in the Fall Classic didn't come around until 1971. I loved daytime World Series games. It was like having a national holiday that was just so special for those who either attended the games or watched them on television. The last daytime World Series game was in 1987, and I truly believe the Major Leagues should mix in a day game or two now—at least on the weekends. I realize the television networks run everything, and rightfully so, with all the money they pay for the rights, but I think day games in the World Series would be great for the future of the game so more fans—especially children—could stay up and watch them until the end.

Under a steady drizzle, Game 1 began as a pitcher's duel between Tiant and Gullett. Neither team—with great hitting on both sides—could plate a run as the game moved to our bottom half of the seventh inning. Then the flood gates opened for us. Luis, who had been untouchable on the mound at Fenway for a month—not allowing an earned run there for 36 innings through this game—showed he could still hit, as well, and got our six-run winning rally started with a single to left, his first base hit since October 3, 1972. Because of the designated hitter rule that was enacted in the American League in 1973, it had been three years since Tiant came to bat—and now, with warm-up jacket on, his memorable and comical adventures around the bases would begin.

I came up to the plate next and dropped a bunt up the first base line. Gullett fielded it and, looking to get the sliding, lead-running Tiant out at second, threw the ball into centerfield. Luis picked himself off the ground and started running to third, then realized he'd be a dead duck and scampered back into second base barely ahead of Geronimo's throw behind him. It was all Luis Tiant's personality—like, *Oops, I've got to get back!*

Denny Doyle, after failing to sacrifice us into scoring position, singled past shortstop to load the bases. Yaz then followed with a soft liner to Griffey in right field that dropped at his feet. Luis, who thought it might be caught, had to hustle back to third to tag up and then run as hard as he could to score. After initially missing home plate, Tiant scrambled back to touch it, and we had a 1–0 lead. On the bench after his baserunning exploits, poor Luis needed oxygen to catch his breath. But his escapades on the basepaths only served to enhance the legend of El Tiante in the annals of baseball lore.

Gullett's day was over, but our rally continued against the Reds' bullpen, and we would add five more runs to take a 6–0 lead. It would be all the runs we would need as Luis continued his mastery over the Big Red Machine. With the crowd chanting, "Loo-ey, Loo-ey, Loo-ey" and his charismatic father Luis Sr. watching proudly from the stands, Tiant retired the Reds in order in the eighth and ninth innings to seal our victory. El Tiante stole the show in Game 1 and proved once more what a true treasure he was to baseball. It was a privilege to play with him and to watch him during one of the greatest times I had in the game.

Inclement weather continued in Game 2, with wind, rain, cold temperatures, and a playing field drenched under a couple of inches of water. But we had a job to do and didn't let our surroundings affect our game. Like in Game 1, it was another pitcher's duel into the late innings, this time between Jack Billingham and Bill Lee.

We held a 2–1 lead into the ninth inning with Lee, still on the hill, having allowed just four hits. Lee had baffled the Reds all afternoon, mixing his full arsenal of pitches including the "Leephus Pitch," his personalized variation of the eephus pitch. But a rain delay that lasted half an hour after the top of the seventh and caused Lee to sit for as long as he did had an adverse effect on him and, despite pitching a scoreless eighth, he was hit hard.

Clinging to a one-run lead to start the ninth, Bench led off and slapped a Lee screwball toward me down the line in right field for a double. It was a real good piece of hitting, as Bench stayed back on the ball very well. Darrell Johnson pulled Lee from the game and replaced him with Dick Drago—a move that Lee, to this day, believes was a big mistake. Lee notes how Drago was up three times in the bullpen—in the fifth, seventh, and ninth innings— and was gassed. Bill contends that Roger Moret would have been a much better option and should have actually started the ninth inning, as Lee was tired. But his biggest complaint was over Johnson not going out for a mound visit in the eighth to check on him after the Reds belted two rockets off him. I don't question Bill because he was such a great athlete and competitor—and he listened to what his body was telling him. But as a 23-year-old, I also wasn't going to question Johnson for leaving Lee in there. People can question Johnson's managing all they want in that situation, but if I couldn't have Tiant in his prime, Lee was the guy

I wanted on the mound because of his competitive nature. With Lee, you never worried much about him allowing runners to get on base. Many times, he would win 2–1 or 3–2 games and give up 11 hits because he would pick a guy off, get a key double play, or induce a pop up just at the right time. That was Lee's game. And he could field his position with the best of them.

Drago started his relief stint well, retiring the first two batters—Perez and Foster—and we were just one out away from taking a 2–0 lead in the World Series. With the Fenway Faithful on their feet, Concepcion hit a hopper up the middle that Doyle got to, but he couldn't make the throw to first and the game was tied at 2–2. After Concepcion stole second, Griffey doubled him home with a drive to deep left center to give the Reds the lead. We went down quietly in the bottom of the ninth and, instead of going up two games, the Series was now tied at one game apiece. However, instead of thinking about what could have been, all I was thinking was, *Tough loss, but you can't worry about what happened. We move on to the next game.*

The next three games moved to Cincinnati, where the Reds had dominated the regular season and NLCS with a remarkable 64–17 record (.795 winning percentage). Their home record that season remains the best ever by a National League team.

In Game 3, they looked to continue their supremacy at Riverfront Stadium, coming out swinging with home runs from Bench, Concepcion, and Geronimo off Rick Wise to take a 5–1 lead after five innings. But we battled back, and when Bernie Carbo hit a pinch-hit solo homer in the seventh, we had cut their lead in half. The Reds remained out in front 5–3 heading into the top of the ninth. After Lynn struck out to start the frame, Petrocelli singled to bring me up to bat as the tying run. Sparky Anderson, as he often did, changed pitchers—bringing in their closer Rawly Eastwick to face me. I hit a 1-0 high and inside fastball—right in my wheelhouse—deep over the left field fence to tie the game at 5–5. It was the biggest moment of my short baseball career and helped force extra innings. Winning even one game in Cincinnati and forcing the series to return to Boston was immensely important to us.

After we failed to score in the top of the tenth, Jim Willoughby returned to the mound for his fourth inning of relief. Willoughby had been sensational, pitching to the minimum nine Reds hitters he faced out of the bullpen. But Geronimo would lead off the Reds' 10th with a single, and it would set up the most controversial play of the World Series. Ed Armbrister came up to pinch hit for Eastwick and squared around to sacrifice Geronimo to second. After Armbrister bunted the ball on one bounce directly in front of home plate, Fisk grabbed it but got tangled up with Armbrister as he attempted to throw Geronimo out at second. As a result, Fisk's throw sailed past Rick Burleson into center field to give the Reds second and third and nobody out. According to the rule book, if Armbrister impeded Fisk from making a throw down to second, what should have occurred was for Armbrister to be called out for interference with Geronimo forced back to first base. Whether it was truly interference or not, I don't know. Unfortunately for us, home plate umpire Larry Barnett didn't think so, and the play stood. After Moret intentionally walked Rose to load the bases, he struck out pinch-hitter Merv Rettenmund for the first out of the inning, giving us hope we could somehow get out of the inning. But it wasn't to be, as Morgan drove home the winning run with a single to center to give the Reds a 6–5 victory.

It was my career in a nutshell. I hit a huge home run off Eastwick to tie a World Series game in the ninth inning—and was really excited about it—but the non-interference call completely overshadowed what would have been a nice moment personally. The Armbrister play was all anyone wanted to talk about after the game, and rightfully so, but it's just the way things always worked out for me.

In Game 4, Tiant again showed what he was made of as one of the great competitors in the game. He wasn't nearly as sharp as he had been over the last six weeks, but he pitched what may have been his most gutsy performance of the year. Luis ended up throwing 155 pitches, and despite the Reds having had two runners on base in four of the last five innings, he held on for a 5–4 complete game victory to tie the series at two games each.

Just like in the two previous games, the drama went right down to the final inning. In this one, as we clung to a 5–4 lead in the ninth, Geronimo led off the bottom of the inning with a single, then was moved to second on a sacrifice bunt (this time with no signs of interference!) by Armbrister. After Rose walked to put the potential winning run on first, Johnson came out to the mound to check on Luis. Tiant told him, "This is *my* game. Get out of here. Get your butt back in the dugout."

Griffey, the next Reds' next hitter, would drive a 3-2 pitch deep to left center field that appeared to be a bases-clearing game-winner for the Reds. But Lynn raced back toward the wall at full speed, extended his glove as far as it could reach, and made a tremendous over-the-shoulder catch for the second out.

We still weren't out of the woods with would-be National League MVP Morgan coming to the plate. The tension remained high with Tiant trying to record the final out. With both Drago and Jim Burton ready to come in from the bullpen, there was little doubt, at this point, that Johnson was sticking with Tiant until the very end—for better or worse. After serving the first pitch wild high, Luis got Morgan to pop up to Yaz at first base to end the game.

Yaz took a big hop and raced toward Tiant in exultation and with a tremendous sense of relief. I hustled in from right field to join the celebration, and the first teammate to embrace me was Yaz. It was a great moment in time.

Personally, I was really locked in at the plate. Trailing 2–0 in the third, I tripled to right field to score two runs to tie the game. It also helped ignite a five-run rally that inning that would give us all the runs we would need to defeat the Reds. I later singled and just missed hitting a home run with a deep drive to center in the eighth.

I truly loved being in the World Series. I loved the elements of the heightened pressure, excitement, and what we all dreamed it to be as kids. And here I was in that situation—and making the most of it. I think my concentration level in the World Series (in both '75 and later in '86) was so much higher than usual, and I often asked myself why I couldn't achieve that same concentration level at other times. I still don't know why I couldn't. But being in the World Series was the ultimate dream of being in the major leagues, and to respond as well as I did to the kind of pressure it produced was something I will never forget.

Game 5 was all about the performance of two of the Reds' biggest stars—Gullett and Pérez. Gullett had a two-hitter through 8⅔ innings before surrendering three straight hits and getting lifted for Eastwick with two outs. Eastwick would strike out Petrocelli to end the game and secure a 6–2 Reds victory, giving them a 3–2 edge in the Series. And Pérez would break out of an 0-for-15 start to the series by hitting two long home runs—a solo shot in the fourth and a three-run blast in the sixth—off Reggie Cleveland.

In my mind, Tony Pérez was one of the true leaders on the Reds and kept that Big Red Machine of theirs running. The biggest mistake the Reds made was trading him to Montreal after the following season. They didn't win with the core of that great team again after Tony left the club.

With the Reds leading the Series three games to two, we would return to Boston to play Game 6. But it rained, and then it rained some more, and it continued to rain after that. What would turn out to be the greatest game in baseball history was delayed three days by rain. But for the fans and players alike, the wait would be worth it. The first five games, with all their majesty, would turn out to be an appetizer for the main course that was to come.

Our World Series had captured the imagination of the country and brought the game's popularity back after several years of malaise. Football had become king, with baseball being seen more and more as a sedentary sport by comparison. Yet our series against the Reds had been so riveting that more than 70 million viewers would tune in to Game 6 on television, easily blowing past the previous record.

The rainouts between the fifth and sixth games certainly increased the drama and anxiousness we all felt, but the inactivity also led to concerns of coming out stale. I never liked having even one day off, much less three, for that very reason. One positive was that the rainouts allowed Johnson to come back with the now immortalized Tiant—who had already beaten the Reds twice—on full rest and move Lee to pitch a potential seventh game. While this didn't sit well with Lee, you couldn't blame Johnson for making the move in a must-win scenario for us.

Another positive was that it allowed Lynn to get some much-needed rest. The last third of the season, Lynn wasn't hitting for power much at all. His weight had dropped to just 170 pounds after playing the most games—both minor and major leagues—of his career that year. So, when he came to the ballpark before Game 6, he had more energy than he'd had in quite some time.

The rest paid immediate dividends for Lynn when he belted a long three-run home run 20 rows beyond the right-center-field bullpen to give us a 3–0 lead in the first inning. It felt great to have that lead, especially with our ace on the mound that night.

The score remained 3–0 until the fifth inning, when the Reds put together a rally to knot the game at 3–3. But it could have been far worse. After a one-out walk to Armbrister, Rose followed with a single to put Reds on the corners. That's when Griffey drove one deep to center field at the 379-foot marker that Lynn leaped for, his shoulder and back crashing hard against the concrete portion of the wall. As Lynn sort of crumpled to the ground motionless, I raced over to retrieve the ball and fired it back into the infield. Armbrister and Rose would both score with Griffey reaching third base with a triple to cut our lead to 3–2. Yaz and I were the first to arrive at Lynn's side and it looked serious. First of all, when you hit concrete, it's very painful—especially when you have the momentum going into it like Lynn had on that play. And secondly, it's always concerning when one of your premier players goes down and you must try to figure out how you're going to replace him.

With Johnson and our trainer Charlie Moss around Lynn, Yaz and I moved off to the side just hoping that Freddie would be alright. The crowd was eerily quiet with the belief that Lynn was knocked out. But he never lost consciousness. What happened was that he lost all feeling from the waist down and was afraid to move. Initially, he thought he broke his back. But then Lynn started to get a tingly feeling like when you hit your funny bone. That was a good sign. Then he started moving around to see if all his other body parts were working, including his legs. When his legs started moving, his football background from USC kicked in and he said, "Okay, I'm alright," and was suddenly back on his feet. The crowd cheered with a sense of relief. As his teammates, there was no better feeling than to see him stay in the game. He meant so much to us and was such a great player.

Despite the Reds being back in the game, we felt fortunate that Lynn was not seriously injured. The next year, the Red Sox would put padding on the wall.

Tiant would retire the next hitter, Morgan, for the second out, but then Bench slammed a single off the wall to score Griffey to tie it up. The Reds ended Tiant's streak of 40 consecutive scoreless innings in Fenway Park that inning. The Big Red Machine was just too talented and astute not to adjust to Tiant, especially when facing him for the third time in the series. The more pitches you see against a certain hitter, the better educated you become when facing him.

The score remained deadlocked until the seventh when Foster belted a two-out, two-run double to center field to give the Reds a 5–3 lead. An inning later, Geronimo made it 6–3 with a solo shot right down the right-field line that would end Tiant's night. With our ace now out of the game and down three runs, we were pretty discouraged but not demoralized. We knew we needed to come back quickly.

In our half of the eighth, Lynn—bouncing back nicely from his back and shoulder injury—got a rally of our own going by lining a single off Pedro Borbon's leg. Petrocelli followed with a walk to bring the tying run to the plate with nobody out. Anderson had seen enough and brought in his closer Eastwick to face me. I had taken Eastwick deep in Game 3, but the result would be different this time, with Rawly getting his revenge by striking me out on a 3-2 pitch. After Burleson lined out to short for the second out, we were just four outs away from elimination.

But when Bernie Carbo was sent to the plate to pinch hit for
Moret, it would set up one of the greatest moments in baseball
history. Bernie already had a pinch-hit home run in Game 3 and
we were praying he could repeat the feat now in this huge spot.
Eastwick's strategy was to mainly pound the zone with inside fastballs on Carbo's hands and he managed to work the count to 2-2.
After the game, Carbo would say how all he kept telling himself
was, "Don't strike out." Eastwick delivered another inside fastball
and Carbo took one of the ugliest defensive swings I had ever
seen—like a little leaguer—but managed to get a piece of it to
stay alive. Bernie was a tremendous ballplayer who had been the
Reds' No. 1 draft choice in 1965—ahead of Bench—but for him
to come off the bench in that situation was extremely difficult. So,
for him to get a piece of that nasty fastball—even while looking
bad doing it—was quite a feat. Still, he looked overmatched against
Eastwick. Now, I wouldn't have bet a million dollars against what
was about to come next, but after seeing Carbo's horrible swing,
I was almost in shock to see him turn on an Eastwick high and
inside fastball and crush it deep into the centerfield bleachers for
a three-run homer to tie the game at 6–6! Carbo jumped for joy
and practically floated around the bases before we mobbed him
in the dugout.

I have long said that the biggest home run I ever saw was the
one that Dave Henderson hit for us 11 years later in the 1986
ALCS, but the second biggest was this one by Carbo. None of the
heroics that were still to come in that game would have happened
if Bernie didn't hit that home run. It just energized us and brought
the team back from the dead. The timing, the moment, it was just
a tremendous boost. When I later watched a highlight film of the
'75 World Series at Fenway, narrator Joe Garagiola couldn't have
described the end of Carbo's at bat any better, saying, "He went

from having the worst swing of the World Series to one of the best swings of the World Series."

At this point, we knew we were playing in a game for the ages. Earlier in the contest—even *before* Carbo's dramatic home run—I was standing on third and Rose came over to me, looked directly in my eyes, and said, "Dewey, isn't this an unbelievable game? This might be the *greatest* game I've ever played in. Can you believe we're playing in this game?" I was only 23 and just excited to even be in a World Series, so I didn't have the whereabouts to look around and realize how great the game was. But when Rose said that, I started looking around at the crowd and it was like an awakening in me. I thought, *Oh, Pete Rose just said this might be the greatest game he had ever played in. Pete Rose!* It was at that moment that I realized the magnitude of it all.

A few words on Rose. Pete is a true treasure of baseball and I believe he belongs in the Hall of Fame. Rose is a flawed individual with a gambling addiction. And I realize he broke the cardinal sin of betting on baseball while manager of the Reds (wagering on his club to win each time). But Major League Baseball now has partnerships with sports betting companies, making its hardline stance on Rose somewhat hypocritical. Additionally, there may very well be players today in the Hall of Fame who broke other rules of the game—including steroid use—but were never caught. I would love to see Commissioner Manfred make an all-out effort to give renewed Hall of Fame consideration to Pete Rose while he is alive by at least allowing his name to be put on the ballot.

Bernie's blast turned the momentum of the game in our favor, and we loaded the bases with nobody out in the bottom of the ninth. Victory was at hand, we believed. But unfortunately, we would be doomed by some miscommunication on the base paths. Lynn hit a short fly ball to left field—more like a 170-foot *pop-up*—to Foster. Doyle, our runner on third, tagged up, thinking he heard our third base coach Zimmer tell him, "Go! Go! Go!" But what Zim was really saying was, "No! No! No!" With all the crowd noise and excitement of the moment, that confusion can happen, and I never blamed either one of them. Watching Doyle hustle down the third base line, the only hope we had was that the throw would be off. But Foster's throw to Bench was perfect and Doyle was out by a mile. Petrocelli followed with a groundout to third and that was the end of our threat. A golden opportunity was missed. The game would go into extra innings with the momentum shifting once again—this time the Reds' way.

After both clubs went down quietly in the 10th, Rose led off the 11th being hit by a pitch. After Griffey's sacrifice bunt attempt was foiled by Fisk throwing out the lead runner Rose at second, Morgan came to bat with one out and one on.

This would set the stage for the signature defensive play of my career. With Morgan, a left-handed batter at the plate, I lined myself up with the foul pole. That's because every time a left-handed hitter hits a ball, whether it's down the left-field line or the right-field line, the ball tends to curve slightly toward the lines. With Morgan, I wasn't only anticipating a line drive base hit directly at me, but also a ball in the gap, a ball down the line, a ground ball in the hole, and a ball hit over my head to my right or to my left. And since there's no tomorrow, I've got to be willing to go into the stands, too. All these scenarios went through my mind between pitches.

I also watched closely where Fisk was setting up for Dick Drago's pitches. Fisk was great at moving around behind the plate. He would fake setting up inside and then go outside or fake outside and come back inside. The hitter couldn't cheat with Fisk moving around like that, so by watching him and where he ended it, I knew where the pitch was going to be thrown. I also relied on Doyle at second to give me a signal as to what pitch was coming.

So, I was well-prepared to anticipate where the ball might be hit to me.

Morgan would smash a 1-1 pitch directly over my head in right field. My first instinct was to turn to my left and run toward the fence. I ran that way because I anticipated the ball was going to curve that way. But as I got closer to the warning track, the ball never broke—it stayed straight, which is so rare. Morgan had hit down on the ball, so it didn't hook and didn't have the spin on it like it usually would. Once I got to the warning track—not aware of where the fence was—I tried drifting back to get in line with the ball, but I lost its arc for a split second, which is a horrible feeling. You always want to see the ball coming into your glove when you are about to catch it. But I jumped for the ball—arching my back—threw my glove up and caught it behind my head by my left shoulder. No one was more surprised than me when it landed in my glove. It was such an awkward catch that I was amazed I caught it. I can't say if I took a home run away from Morgan, but it was close.

Meanwhile, Griffey was nearly all the way to third and had to hustle back to first base. Looking to double him up, I regained my footing, turned myself around, and the first thing I saw were the lights above third base. It was like looking into the sun for a second. I was kind of blinded by them, so I just threw the ball in the general direction of first base. The throw was off, but Yaz had plenty of time to field it near where the grass meets the coaches' box and toss it to Burleson who came over to cover first base to complete the double play for the third out.

After the game, my catch was already being compared with other great World Series catches like Willie Mays' over-the-shoulder one in 1954 and Al Gionfriddo's robbing Joe DiMaggio of a home run in 1947. Sparky Anderson told reporters that night, "That's the best catch I've seen. We'll never see one any better." If

I hadn't made that catch, Griffey would have easily scored, and Morgan would have been, at a minimum, in scoring position with just one out, setting the Reds up for a World Series victory. I've always said it wasn't the greatest catch I ever made, but it was, without question, the *most important* one.

This epic game was still tied at 6–6 well past midnight and had lasted more than four hours. It was now time for one last bit of theatrics as Fisk came to the plate to face Pat Darcy, the eighth Reds pitcher Anderson used. The situation was a good one for Carlton—a lowball, dead-pull hitter against a lowball pitcher. On Darcy's second pitch, a low inside sinker, Fisk sent a line drive high and straight down the line in left field toward the Green Monster. As Fisk stood a few feet up the first base line, he famously waved his arms to his right—using body English to try to keep the ball from going foul. On the bench, we were all kind of doing the same—angling ourselves for the ball to *stay fair, stay fair, stay fair!* And thankfully, Fisk had hit it so hard, and on a line, that it didn't have a chance to hook. He always worked so hard on hitting down on the ball to get a back spin—and that's exactly what he did here. So, it wasn't surprising that when he hit Darcy's pitch, it wasn't hooking too much. The ball would slam against the mesh attached to the foul pole for a game-winning home run for the ages—one of the most cherished moments in baseball history.

As I look back at that truly historic game, taking nothing away at all from how big Fisk's home run was, I think Carbo's homer was even bigger. While Fisk's is the most celebrated in Red Sox history, if Bernie doesn't hit that home run, I don't make my game-saving catch and Carlton doesn't hit that walk-off home run. Carbo made all the dramatics that would come later possible.

It was the end of the most emotional game I had ever played in. The back-and-forth was what made the game so special right to the end. And most importantly, we had lived for another day, as there would be a Game 7 in this remarkable World Series.

Game 7 often gets overlooked because of how incredible Game 6 was, but the final game of the '75 Series was a thriller in its own right. The hype going in was unreal, as it may have been the most highly anticipated World Series game ever. It would attract a television audience of 75,900,000—the largest of all time. But despite all that was on the line, we were focused and as loose as we could be under the circumstances. And that included Bill Lee, our starting pitcher that night. After hearing Sparky Anderson tell reporters during the pregame press conference, "No matter what the outcome of this game, [starting pitcher] Don Gullett is going to the Hall of Fame," Lee, as only he could, quipped, "No matter what happens in this game, I'm going to the *Eliot Lounge!*"

Just like in Game 6, we jumped out to an early 3–0 lead. Gullett was wild and issued a one-out walk to Carbo to start our rally in the third inning. After Doyle singled, Yaz ripped an RBI single to right field to give us a 1–0 lead. On the play, after the throw went into third base, Yaz astutely advanced to second to give us runners in scoring position. Fisk was intentionally walked to load the bases and, after Lynn struck out, Gullett walked Petrocelli to give us a 2–0 edge. That brought me to the plate with a chance to really break the game open early. Even at the young age of 23, there was no panic in me over the magnitude of the situation. I showed patience looking for a certain pitch in a particular area and stayed true to that strategy. One thing I wasn't afraid of was striking out because, when you are, you often do exactly that. By being patient without fear of striking out, it allows you to go deeper into counts and see more pitches. And the more pitches you see, the more education you have as a hitter.

As it turned out, Gullett didn't give me anything close to hit—walking me on four pitches—and our lead increased to 3–0. Burleson struck out to end the inning, but we were off to the best start we could have imagined. We had the Reds' ace pitcher on the ropes while we had one of the best money pitchers in the game—cool and confident Lee—successfully using his hard screwball, sinker, the occasional Leephus pitch, and everything else in his arsenal to keep the Cincinnati hitters off-balance.

With Anderson's "Hall of Fame pitcher" Gullett long gone from the game, Lee was cruising—protecting our 3–0 lead into the top of the sixth. But with two outs and a man on, Pérez was ready for the Leephus pitch and crushed it over the Green Monster to cut our lead to 3–2. Pérez was such a great hitter that he was able to take a stride and then—because the eephus is so slow—come back with his left foot, re-stride, and time the pitch perfectly. Lee has been second-guessed over the years for throwing that pitch in that situation, but I don't question it. Pérez could have just as easily popped it up, grounded out, or hit a foul ball. You've just got to give credit to the guy that hit it out of the park. No one, that I can recall, had ever taken that pitch deep against Lee.

We were still clinging to a 3–2 lead in the top of the seventh when, with one out, Lee uncharacteristically walked Griffey on four pitches. As it turned out, Lee had developed a blister on his throwing hand and was relieved by Moret. It was a daunting assignment for any reliever in such a high-stakes game, much less a young pitcher like Moret, and after issuing a two-out walk to Armbrister, Rose singled to center to tie the game at 3–3. It was just one more time in this remarkable World Series when a team came from behind to tie it. But we had great players that stayed calm under tough situations like this one. We never got too high or too low throughout the ebbs and flows of the series, always remaining on an even keel. Moret giving up that tying base hit to Rose—a guy that squared up a baseball more times than anybody ever in baseball history—was just part of the game.

After Moret walked Morgan to load the bases, Johnson replaced him with Jim Willoughby, who proceeded to retire Bench to end the inning and prevent any more damage. After we were retired in the bottom of the seventh, Willoughby went back out and pitched a perfect eighth, setting the Reds down in order. Willoughby looked sensational. In our half of the eighth, I led off the inning with a walk, but Burleson couldn't sacrifice me to second and, with two strikes, hit into a double play. Then, in a move that would be debated in Boston for years to come, Johnson pinch-hit Willoughby for Cecil Cooper, who was in the midst of a 1-for-18 slump. What made the move so controversial was that Willoughby was dealing and was likely the best option to keep the Reds in check in the ninth. But I fully supported Johnson's move because, even though Cooper was slumping, Cecil was on his way to becoming one of the best hitters in baseball history. He could just flat-out hit. You can't even consider that he was in a slump at the time. Instead, you look at a guy like Cooper and think he's due to break out. So, I would take those odds any day of the week with a hitter like Cecil hitting over Willoughby in that situation. The other thing was that Johnson probably didn't want the Reds to have the chance to see Willoughby go around their lineup a second time.

As it turned out, Cooper ended the inning by popping out to Rose at third, setting the stage for this World Series to go down to the final inning with the score still tied at three apiece. It simply *had* to come down to this.

Johnson brought Jim Burton in to pitch the ninth—another move I can't put down. After yielding a couple of walks but getting

two men out, Morgan singled home the go-ahead run with a
blooper off the end of his bat to give the Reds a 4-3 lead. Of
course, all the Boston talk shows afterward were screaming, *"How
can you bring in Jim Burton?!"* But what if Burton got through
that inning? Would it still have been talked about? No, of course
not. The manager must trust and use his entire team. If Johnson
didn't have confidence in Burton, he would never have put him
out there. So, Burton was the right guy in the right spot. It just
turned out that you've got a round ball and a round bat and, even
though Morgan didn't square it up and hit it off the end of the
bat, it still dropped in for a bloop single. It happens. It's so easy
for the talking heads and the writers to second guess.

After Reggie Cleveland came in to retire Pérez to end the top
of the ninth, we still had a chance for a dramatic climax to this
majestic World Series. But we went down quietly, with Yaz ending
it by flying out to Geronimo in center field. The closeness of this
pristine Fall Classic had come down to an end-of-the-bat bloop
single. The history books would show just how close it was over
the seven-game series—we had a total of 60 hits to the Reds' 59,
and we had 30 runs to the Reds' 29. But the Big Red Machine did
what it did best—they won when it counted most.

Despite how much it hurt to lose a World Series that was as
close as this one, at the time I was very bullish on the future.
I figured with the team we had, we would be in three or four
World Series over the next five years. Unfortunately, in part due
to the changing tide in baseball's economic system, it wouldn't
turn out that way. The greatest World Series would be the last
pure World Series.

CHAPTER 9

A WHOLE NEW BALLGAME

SHORTLY AFTER THE WORLD SERIES ENDED, Susan and I welcomed our daughter, Kirstin, into the world. Our deep concerns over whether she—like her brother Timothy—would be born with NF proved unwarranted. Thank God she was born healthy, and that NF never moved on to her. She is, to this day, fine as far as that goes—a true blessing.

On the baseball front, I was still basking in the glow from the excitement of the Red Sox winning the pennant and taking the Reds down to the final inning of a classic World Series that captured the imagination of the entire sports world. And although I never sought or relished the spotlight, my clutch hitting and the catch I made in Game 6 of the Fall Classic propelled me into the conversation as one of the top outfielders in the game. I didn't want the headlines and never sought any attention, but I knew I was a better player than some people on the talk shows and in the newspapers gave me credit for prior to the World Series. Now all that had changed.

With a full year of Jim Rice, Fred Lynn, and Carlton Fisk and the additions of future Hall of Fame pitcher Ferguson Jenkins and reliever Tom House, we were heavy favorites to repeat as division champions. If anything, we were even stronger than the year before and felt there was no way any club was going to keep us from going back to the World Series in the years ahead. But 1976 would remarkably be the beginning of the "dynasty that never was." With the core of our team intact over the next three seasons, it still totally boggles my mind to this day that we would not return to the World Series.

There were major distractions at play at the outset of the '76 season, which played heavily with the chemistry of the club. Salary disputes involving Fisk, Burleson, and Lynn were at the forefront—and there were even rumors that Freddie might get traded to the Angels if he didn't sign soon. All of this came on the heels of pitchers Andy Messersmith of the Dodgers and Dave McNally of the Expos not signing their 1975 contracts and becoming free agents after arbitrator Peter Seitz ruled they were no longer bound to their teams for eternity—effectively killing the reserve clause in baseball and ushering in the free agent era. The decision had a huge impact on the game's landscape. The days of general managers solely building their organizations through the farm system and trades was over.

Lynn, Burleson, and Fisk were all clients of agent Jerry Kapstein and went into the '76 season unsigned because they had the foresight to believe that the Messersmith–McNally case was going to be won and that free agency was going to happen. At a minimum, they would have some bargaining power and, if necessary, they could walk and become free agents themselves. There was a real possibility of them playing elsewhere less than one year removed from our glorious '75 campaign.

During those early days of free agency, agents were not very popular at all, with the perception by many that they were going to destroy baseball. So, a guy like Kapstein had some very good players and the power to manipulate the game. There were so many uncertainties and unanswered questions. *How are teams going to manage? How are the owners going to make any money? How will the small-market teams survive?*

I would get an agent myself the next year, because the owners almost made it so that you *had* to have one. There was just no way that a player could go in and talk himself up in negotiating a new contract. And if you had a big enough ego and tried, I don't know if a team would really want somebody like that. But to have an agent say all the right things for you and compare you to other players was a significant advantage at the bargaining table.

It was a far cry from how contracts were done just a couple of years before. After the '74 season, I went into general manager Dick O'Connell's office to negotiate my own deal. For comparison's sake, I brought up Garry Maddox, a centerfielder with the San Francisco Giants, whom I likened myself to because he played great defense and could hit as well. Maddox was making $50,000, so I asked for the same. O'Connell responded by telling me a story about Australia that went on for about 15 minutes and then, at the end of his story, said, "Okay." I looked at him and said, "What do you mean, 'Okay?' Okay, what?" He said, "Okay, you got your fifty grand." But he had to tell that story about Australia and a trip he took. All the while, I was thinking, *What the heck? Where are we going with this story?* But it was kind of neat, too, because you could go in and you had that rapport with the general manager where it was more personal. With an agent, it became *impersonal.*

In fact, the situation escalated to becoming like a war between the owners and the players and created a very unhealthy environment. It also created a need for agents because the owners would try to take advantage of the players all the time during this period. It was the first time any baseball player ever had anything to say about what happened to him, which was a great thing. Bill Lee called free agency our Emancipation Proclamation and he was right. Everybody else in the country had it but us. Before free agency, fans of a team would see the same players at the same positions for years because they couldn't move to another team. The players basically took what the owners gave them. Even if you were a great player, you might have a little leverage, but not much. But now, it was a brand-new ballgame. If guys like the three we had were unsigned, it was a precursor to all kinds of possibilities.

While I certainly observed what was going on at the dawn of free agency, my focus financially was on completing my fifth year in the big leagues so I would be eligible to receive a pension. Despite my performance in the '75 campaign, there was still some instability in my life. The talk shows and newspapers were regularly talking about the possibility of the Red Sox trading me. Rumors had me going to Milwaukee for third baseman Don Money or Minnesota for pitcher Bert Blyleven. And although the rumors were likely unfounded, it played on my mind as a 23-year-old who recently bought his first house, had just become a father of a second child, and had a son with serious health problems.

As a professional, despite the backdrop of free agency, player holdouts, and trade rumors, my focus was on helping a great Red Sox team get back into the World Series. But the off-field distractions were very real, and we started off the '76 season terribly with a 6–15 record—which included a 10-game losing streak. We had a team batting average of just .256 and a staff ERA of 4.60. There was a malaise over the club, and we were making mental mistakes uncharacteristic of our group.

———————

It was still early in the season with plenty of time to turn things around but, of course, the Boston media was all over our slow start. One local television station brought a Salem witch to Fenway to try to exorcise the demons. They went to Fisk to see if he would participate, and I remember him being pretty upset over the whole thing. I didn't care for the stunt, either, but I wasn't as boisterous about it. I didn't like the microphone, anyway, and the less I said the better it was. So they went to Bernie Carbo, who was more than willing to allow them to put the witch's hat on his head. The press made a big deal out of it, but it really was a non-event and meant nothing to me. We were too good of a team and soon got hot with improved pitching and hitting—certainly not because of a Salem witch examining our auras.

We would win seven of eight games prior to going to New York on May 20 to begin a critical four-game series against the first-place Yankees, cutting their lead over us from 8½ games down to six in the process. For an early season series, there was an electricity in the air, and the first game would exemplify the intensity of our rivalry with the Yankees over the next three years.

With the Yankees leading 1–0 with two outs and runners on first and second in the sixth, Otto Velez lined a one-hopper to me in right field. I came up firing and delivered a perfect throw to Fisk ahead of a charging Lou Piniella by at least 15 feet. Piniella tried to jar the ball out of Fisk's catcher's mitt with his forearm but missed the glove and got him in the head, setting off a huge brawl at home plate. This was a serious brawl, unlike so many you see today where there's just a lot of pushing, shoving, and wrestling. Fisk came up punching Piniella, while Mickey Rivers hit Lee—our starting pitcher that night—in the back of the head before Graig Nettles dumped Spaceman on his left shoulder by the first base line. Lee, who won 17 games for us in each of the previous three seasons, suffered a separated shoulder in the melee. Despite this, just as it seemed the brawl was over, Lee went over to Nettles and screamed something at him before Graig popped him right in the mouth, and the fight was on again. Rivers was going around sucker-punching some of our guys in the back of the head, which we didn't appreciate. When Lee got back up off the ground again, his left arm hung like a spaghetti noodle, and he was helped back into the dugout by our trainer Charlie Moss to the delight of the Bronx crowd. As a result of his injury, Lee would never be able to throw hard again—becoming a junk-baller—and would miss most of the rest of the season. Lee's absence would be a huge loss for us. Tongue-in-cheek, he blames me for the whole ordeal, saying that if I didn't make a perfect throw to Fisk to get Piniella, none of this would have happened to him.

My throw to nail Piniella at the plate was my second assist of the game, as I also threw out Fred Stanley at home to cap an inning-ending double play in the third. There's no question that the strength of my throwing arm was a gift from God. It was not unlike the gift given to a world-class violinist, celloist, or pianist with their respective musical talents. In baseball, it really doesn't matter how big or small or skinny or heavy you are when it comes to God-given talent. I remember standing shoulder-to-shoulder with Don Baylor—who was twice as wide and much stronger than me—and watching him have trouble throwing the ball from left field to second base. By contrast, you look at a guy like Pedro Martínez, who weighed maybe 170 pounds soaking wet but could throw his pitches as hard as anyone. So, arm strength is a gift, but it's a gift that needs to be worked on and developed. Pedro honed his skills—a gift from God that made him elite—by watching others. He particularly loved watching Greg Maddux, one of the smartest pitchers in baseball history, pitch. He wanted to see Maddux—who didn't throw hard at all—so he could learn from him. I did the same, always listening, always learning from others. I can't tell you if I did more arm curls or wrist curls than anybody else, but I worked as hard as I could to get the most out of my strong right arm. And the hard work paid off.

The fight seemed to ignite us, as Burleson homered in the seventh to put us ahead, and Yaz homered twice (borrowing my bat!) in the final two innings to give us an 8–2 victory. "The fight is what did it," Yaz said after the game. "After that we had a will to win I hadn't seen since the World Series. I wasn't just congratulated after the home runs, I was mobbed."

Now just five games out, we had a great opportunity to close the gap in the division, but we dropped back-to-back extra-inning games. In the second game of the series, we couldn't hold a 5–4 lead in the ninth and lost 6–5 in 12 innings when rookie Kerry Dineen, who arrived at Yankee Stadium from Triple-A Syracuse in the *fifth inning*, singled home Carlos May with the winning run. The RBI would represent half of his career total of two—just our luck. The third game of the series was a pitchers' duel between Dick Pole and Catfish Hunter. The game remained scoreless into the bottom of the 11th when May singled home Willie Randolph to give the Yankees a 1–0 victory and increase their division lead to seven games. Catfish was impressive, pitching all 11 innings while giving up just three hits. We usually had success against Hunter (3–0 against him in '75), which made wasting a great effort by Pole and then Tom House all the more brutal. Thankfully, we took the fourth game of the series 7–6 in a contest that saw two ties and four lead changes. After the intense series was over, we left the Bronx the way we came in—six games out.

We would keep pace with the Yankees over the next three weeks, and on the morning of the trading deadline of June 15 we were just five games out. We had arrived in Oakland early that day after a series in Minnesota. None of us could have predicted the craziness that was to come late that afternoon. When the team arrived at the Oakland Coliseum, everybody was buzzing about two moves that A's owner Charlie Finley had just made. Finley sold left fielder Joe Rudi and reliever Rollie Fingers to the Red

Sox for a million dollars each and Vida Blue to the Yankees for
$1.5 million. For Rudi and Fingers, they didn't have to travel very
far to join us. They basically walked over to the visitor's dugout,
suited up in their new Red Sox uniforms, and joined us on the
field before the game. All of us kind of stopped what we were
doing to welcome them. I was thinking, *Well, I don't have to face
Rollie Fingers anymore.* For me, that was the greedy side of a player,
since Fingers was a very talented, special relief pitcher. While I
could certainly understand the interest in acquiring Fingers as our
closer, I wasn't sure where Rudi, a terrific player, was going to fit
in, as our outfield was set with Rice, Lynn, and myself—with Yaz
moving between first and left field. It's possible he would be used
as leverage or insurance in the event Lynn remained unsigned
after the season ended.

As it turned out, neither Fingers or Rudi played a single inning
for us, nor Blue for the Yankees, as Baseball Commissioner Bowie
Kuhn, upon hearing of the deals, froze them until he could consult
with the owners. Ultimately, Kuhn nullified the trades three days
later by invoking the "best interests of baseball" clause. I'm sure he
got a lot of pressure from the other owners saying it wasn't right
how the Red Sox got access to Rudi and Fingers and the Yankees
access to Blue while they were left out in the cold.

There's no telling how picking up players of Fingers' and Rudi's
caliber might have positively affected our fortunes in the pennant
race. But without their services, an abysmal 12–19 record in July
would bury us in the standings—and would cost Darrell Johnson
his job. I thought it was a panic move in firing Johnson with the
team we had and with almost the entire second half left to play.
But Johnson had a drinking problem and would sometimes come
to the ballpark not entirely sober. I've always believed that's what
got him fired. I loved Darrell. He just had a problem. But I give
him credit for straightening himself out and later becoming a

scout for the Mets. The sober Darrell Johnson was a magnificent baseball man and motivator.

Johnson was replaced by Don Zimmer. Zimmer was not only the best third base coach I've ever been around but was also the *greatest* baseball man I've ever known. He took a lot of pressure off his players when he'd tell us things like, "If I give you the hit-and-run or the steal sign and you're thrown out, it's my fault." Zim was trying to create something, putting pressure on the defense. In that respect, he was a good coach. I got to coach alongside him with the Colorado Rockies in 1994 and had a lot of fun with him there.

That being said, he was not a good people person as a manager, which made him very tough to play for. After I was severely beaned behind my left ear in a game in 1978—waking up in a hospital and having my head hurt like it never hurt before—I suffered from vertigo for almost three years. But just six days after the beaning, I was back in right field and anytime I raised my head and looked upwards, the vertigo set in. On this one fly ball to me, I looked up and saw five balls. The actual baseball kind of hit me in the chest and I fumbled it around before it dropped right in front of me. After the inning ended, I came into the dugout and Zim said, "What happened on that play?" I said, "Zim, every time I put my head up, I see five balls." And he said, "Catch the one in the middle!" And then he just walked away. And here's a guy who was also severely beaned as a player, so you would think he would have had some kind of empathy for my situation. But that wasn't what he was about. He was all about results.

That was the difference between Zim as a coach and as a manager. He was tough as a manager but was still a great baseball man. I say that with the utmost respect. I learned more from him than any other manager I ever played for, but he and I didn't always see eye to eye on things. I don't know what it was, but

Zim always wanted to trade me. He treated me very differently as my manager than as a coach. To this day, I have no idea why except that perhaps I wasn't his style of player. Despite his wishes, however, the Red Sox wouldn't trade me. And to his credit, he put my name in the lineup every day.

For as poorly as the '76 campaign was shaping up, at least some consolation was on the way for our future when, in early August, Fisk, Burleson, and Lynn would end their holdouts and would all sign five-year contracts for big money at the time. I wasn't the least bit jealous of their lucrative deals because I knew my time was just around the corner. Most importantly, the dark cloud that hovered over the club for the first four months of the season had finally cleared—even if our season was effectively lost. At least now we could finally get back to just thinking about baseball.

We would finish the year strong, winning 15 of our final 18 games—including a seven-game winning streak in mid-September—which I felt boded well for the '77 season. We never quit and played well under Zim.

After the season, I was awarded my first of eight Gold Glove Awards. I don't know why I wasn't recognized more for the award in either of the previous two years, but maybe the exposure I received in the '75 World Series turned things around for me. But in any event, I never played for awards. With all the talent we still had on the club, I was looking forward to the chance to get back into the postseason in 1977.

CHAPTER 10

THE CRUNCH BUNCH

"**Y**OU'RE *NOT GOING HOME*!" Don Zimmer, the old-school manager, adamantly exclaimed. "Three days away and you're out of shape!" It was the end of spring training in March of '77 and Susan had just gone into labor with our third child, Justin. "Yes, I am, Zim!" I replied sternly, "My wife's in labor. I'll be back tomorrow night, but I've got to be there for my wife." So, without my manager's permission, I drove an hour and fifteen minutes from Winter Haven to Orlando International Airport and caught the next flight up to Boston. The year before we had bought a house in Lynnfield, a suburban town outside of Boston, and to Susan's credit, while she was eight months pregnant, she cared for our two young children while I was down in Florida getting ready for the season.

As soon as I got off the plane at Boston Logan International Airport, I rushed over to a pay phone to call her. She had just given birth to Justin, so like a lot of ballplayers in those days, I wasn't there for the delivery. Back then, I wouldn't have been able to witness the birth unless I had taken numerous courses beforehand, though I could have entered the room immediately afterward. Still, it's a far cry from how maternity leave works now in baseball. If your wife is having a baby, a player can leave the club for three days. I wouldn't want to be out of the game that long and Susan wouldn't expect that, but to try to deprive a player from being with his wife *at all* during this special moment was heartless—especially during *spring training.*

I arrived at the hospital as quickly as I could to be with my wife and newborn son. I was immediately told by the physician that it was a difficult delivery and that Susan almost died on the table. But they were able to revive her and everything was now fine. It was times like these when I wish I had been able to spend more time with my family. But because I was so dedicated to the game—and had to be, for the welfare of my wife and kids—I can't say if it was my fault for not being there more. Still, while I did the best I could, because of my commitment to baseball, I wasn't always the best father or the best husband. The game just took so much time. There's a lot of guilt in me to this day over it all. Sometimes I wish I had decided to become a starting pitcher instead of an every-day player because then I could have had some time for them between starts, but that's not the way it was.

I was extremely fortunate to have a wife who understood the baseball life. There would be many times when I was on the road and Susan was alone with the three kids. She sometimes looked out our living room window and watched our neighbors, Italian immigrants who owned a salon and remain great friends of ours to this day, entertaining family and friends at parties they would host. Sometimes there would be as many as 20 cars in front of their house. By contrast, Susan had no family nearby and two very sick boys and a daughter to care for. So, when I was away with the ball club, she was stuck. She couldn't call her mother, who was living in California, to come over to give her a breather. She never had a breather…*never.* I always recognized this, and it played on me that she didn't have any support while I was away. But she understood that I had to be where I was—playing baseball seven or eight months a year for the Red Sox. Susan is a great person with wonderful character, and I love her dearly.

With Timothy already diagnosed with NF, there was serious concern that Justin might develop the genetic disorder, as well. But at the time of his birth, there were no signs of it in him.

As for Timothy, now almost four years old, we noticed him pulling down his baseball hat to his left side to cover up his puffy left eye. He was beginning to get teased by other kids about it, so this was his way of handling it emotionally. As parents, it was heartbreaking, because we have photos of him before he started doing this and we can see how happy he was. But now that he was getting older, he was becoming more aware of his malady. It was a concern that Susan and I were cognizant of and sensitive to and kept a close watch on in the years to come.

As I'd promised Zim, I flew back down to spring training the next afternoon after Justin's birth. And contrary to what he thought, I was definitely *not* out of shape.

There was a lot of optimism in Red Sox camp that we could reclaim the division throne from the Yankees. During the off-season, we made a splash by signing free-agent reliever Bill Campbell, who was coming off a huge year with the Twins—pitching to a 17–5 record with 20 saves. We also made a trade with the Brewers to re-acquire two familiar faces in Red Sox lore—George "Boomer" Scott and Bernie Carbo—in exchange for Cecil Cooper. It was tough to see a player of Coop's ability leave the club, but he needed to go somewhere else and be his own player. He was always a great hitter, but for some reason he couldn't reach his full potential with the Red Sox. Playing in Boston took a toll on him. Once in Milwaukee, he changed his stance and became like a 6'2" Rod Carew with power. And boy, he really took off, becoming one of the premier first basemen in the game. But I don't blame the Red Sox for trading him. We had too many guys doing the same thing at the first base, left field, and designated hitter positions. Besides, Coop didn't want to DH—he wanted to play in the field—and I don't blame him. But with Yaz and Rice on the club, he just wasn't getting enough opportunities to shine. Cecil was one of the truly great teammates I ever had, and I was so happy that he went on to Milwaukee and was able to show what an extraordinary player he really was. He just needed to go someplace else.

With Boomer, who would exclusively play first base for us, we had another power-hitter to insert into an already lethal lineup. In fact, our '77 lineup was probably the most dangerous the Red Sox ever had. It was so powerful that our No. 8 hitter, third baseman Butch Hobson, hit 30 home runs with 112 RBIs for us that season.

Like others in our lineup, I got off to the best start of my career and, by the end of May, was batting .303 with 11 home runs. But then, on June 1 in a game in Texas, my season came to a crashing halt. I was on first base when Rick Miller doubled to left field. Our third base coach, Eddie Yost, was waving me home. As I came around third, my hamstring popped so loudly it could be heard all the way into the third base dugout. As I successfully scurried back into third, I had no strength at all in my right leg. As a result, my right cleat stayed in the ground—still angled toward home plate. So, as my body turned toward the bag, I tore up the cartilage in my knee.

I immediately had to come out of the game, with Carbo pinch-running and replacing me in right field. Our team physician, Dr. Thomas Tierney, didn't recommend surgery right away. And to be honest, I didn't want it because I was so locked in that season I didn't want to come out of the lineup for an extended period. They didn't have access to MRIs back then to determine exactly how badly I injured myself, but my right knee was like spaghetti—just completely torn up.

I would be out of action for nearly two months—rehabbing as best as I could to get healthy again. But even after my return to the active roster, I played sparingly into August before shutting down for the season. The final straw came when I went into a game and my right knee locked up on me in a 45-degree angle which I couldn't straighten out. I had to leave the game. Inexplicably, Dr. Tierney was angry at me and said curtly, "You need surgery. Come back tomorrow morning and we'll operate on your knee." He wouldn't have lasted very long in today's game.

In my absence, the team continued to bash home runs at a historic rate, finishing the season with 213 dingers, just 27 homers short of the then-record held by the 1961 Yankees. Rice, Scott, and Hobson all finished with more than 30 home runs, with Fisk and Yaz not far behind. Even my replacement, Carbo, contributed 15 homers. We were a run-scoring machine. But most importantly of all, we had the Yankees, who were imploding before our very eyes, on the ropes. In a memorable three-game sweep at Fenway against them in late-June, we pounded out *16* home runs—a major league record for a three-game series—winning by lopsided scores of 9–4, 10–4, and 11–1 to take a 2½-game lead in the Eastern Division.

But it was the second game of the series, a nationally televised Saturday afternoon game on NBC, when the Yankees looked completely cooked. In the bottom of the sixth, we led 7–4 when Rice hit a check-swing fly ball toward Reggie Jackson in right field. But Reggie didn't charge the ball and it dropped in for a base hit. Rice kept running hard and turned his flare into a double. An enraged Yankees manager Billy Martin immediately pulled Jackson from the game for lack of hustle. When Jackson returned to the dugout, Martin was waiting for him, and the two began arguing before Billy lunged at him and had to be restrained by coaches Elston Howard and Yogi Berra. It's probably a good thing for Martin that his coaches stopped him, because Jackson was a lot younger and stronger than he was. I was watching what was unfolding while receiving therapy on my leg and could hardly believe what I was seeing. The Yankees were unraveling both on and off the field for the entire country to see. Martin, who had a notoriously serious drinking problem, was now viewed as a manager who had lost his clubhouse and—with Yankees owner George Steinbrenner en route to Boston—it was widely believed Martin could be fired as early as that evening.

The Yankees weren't the only team we were mashing. Over a 10-game stretch in June, we hit 33 home runs—another major league record. Over the course of the season, we hit five or more home runs in a single game *eight* times, including eight dingers in one game against the Blue Jays. And it wasn't like we were doing this against rookie call-ups. We were taking down future Hall of Famers like Jim Palmer (we had five home runs off him in one game) and Catfish Hunter (four home runs off him in one *inning*). We were just crushing American League pitching no matter who teams threw out there.

At the All-Star Game that July, we sent more representatives—Burleson, Fisk, Lynn, Rice, Scott, Yaz, and Campbell—than any other team. For us, the Midsummer Classic at Yankee Stadium was like a coronation of the remarkable first half of the season we had.

We would hold a 3½-game lead as late as August 18 before the toughest division in baseball tightened up. Not only did the Yankees straighten themselves out (they never did fire Martin) and begin to play like a winner again, but the Orioles were right with us—quietly making a serious bid to win the division themselves.

A brutal and ill-timed seven-game losing streak in late August dropped us two games behind the Yankees and, despite remaining in the thick of the pennant race, we never saw first place again. While we continued to score plenty of runs, we lacked pitching depth, which was exposed when several of our hurlers went down with injuries.

Entering the last weekend of the season, the Yankees, Orioles, and Red Sox were all still in contention. Our mission was simple. We were three games behind the Yankees and had to sweep the Orioles and hope New York would lose all three of their games against Detroit to stay alive. But the Yankees prevailed, winning their 100th game over the Tigers while we split two with the Orioles (the final game was rained out and not made up) and finished with 97 wins.

I truly believe that if both Lynn (torn ligament) and I didn't miss significant playing time, and if Lee—who had to take three cortisone shots for his shoulder that season—was healthier, it would have made up for the 2½ games we finished behind New York. I would have loved an opportunity to see what that outstanding club of ours could have accomplished in the postseason. But injuries are a part of the game, and we'll never know.

CHAPTER 11

THE ONE THAT GOT AWAY

EXPECTATIONS FOR THE 1978 SEASON were soaring. For as strong a team as we had in '77, the trades and signings we made after the season made us an even better, more balanced club. A month after pitching the '77 World Series finale for the Yankees, Mike Torrez—a blood-and-guts "gamer" who hardly ever missed a start—was signed as a free agent and was now in our starting rotation. Two weeks later, we traded for second baseman Jerry Remy, a major upgrade at the position, who could run and hit and would become the sparkplug we needed at the top of our lineup. And then just a week before opening day, we further fortified our pitching staff by trading for Dennis Eckersley, who would win 20 games for us that season and become the ace of the staff. The front office had done a magnificent job in addressing our greatest needs with those acquisitions. To go along with our incredible hitting attack, we had significantly upgraded and deepened our starting rotation, improved our defense, and added more speed. We were built to win—and win big.

In "Eck," I didn't just have a new teammate, but a new friend with whom I hit it off right away. Even years later, after he was traded and I faced him when he was a reliever with Oakland, we were still close. He was trying to get me out and I was trying my best to get a hit off him—there was always a battle, but that friendship remained. That's one of the hardest things about this game. You develop friendships with some of your teammates and then they go to another team. It's a cold game in that respect. That was especially hard for me because I took a friendship very seriously. And Eck, a lifelong friend, was no exception. Luckily, Eck remained in the Boston area for many years after the trade, so we would still see each other, but not as much as I would have liked.

Entering the '78 season, I was excited to be healthy again after busting my rear end the entire winter recovering from knee surgery. I think it made me a better athlete because anytime you get hurt, you must do so much more than your usual exercise routine to get back on the field. And the results reflected that, as I picked up where I left off before my injury—hammering my 15th home run as early as June 17—to go along with a .294 batting average and a .380 OBP. Defensively, the knee injury may have taken 10 percent to 15 percent off my arm strength because I strained to throw off it a bit, but it forced me to use better technique in making more accurate throws and getting rid of the ball quicker. Overall, I had become more efficient using my entire body.

Zim was raving about my performance with the media, saying, "Ten of those [15 home runs] were as long as anybody can hit them." And with my outfield play, Zim told them, "Dewey's always been a great defensive player but even a great defensive player can go all season and not make the kind of throws and catches he did in the last two weeks. He's got third base coaches petrified." Zim even harkened back to his Brooklyn Dodgers days, saying how I had a better throwing arm than their legendary right fielder Carl Furillo, the so-called "Reading Rifle."

Despite all the accolades he bestowed upon me publicly, Zim still wanted to trade me, and I couldn't figure out why. I would listen to the sports talk shows and try to figure out where I was

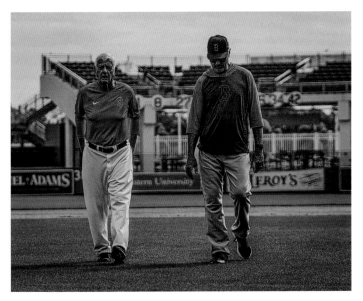

Carl Yastrzemski and me at spring training in 2020 shortly after the passing of my eldest son, Timothy. Yaz lost his son Michael in 2004. Carl and I have a bond that goes well beyond baseball. (Worcester Red Sox)

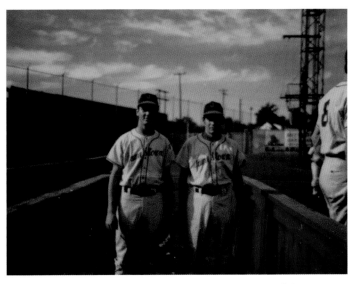

At just 17, I reported to the Jamestown Falcons of the Rookie-Level New York–Penn League. With me was (at right) Freddie Santiago. (Dwight Evans Collection)

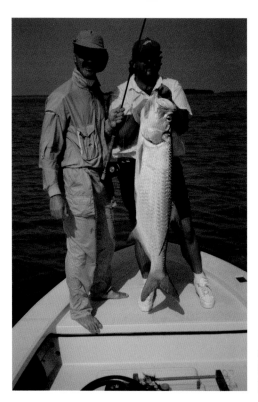

Admiring the 100-pound tarpon I caught fly-fishing at the Florida Keys on my 41st birthday. (Dwight Evans Collection)

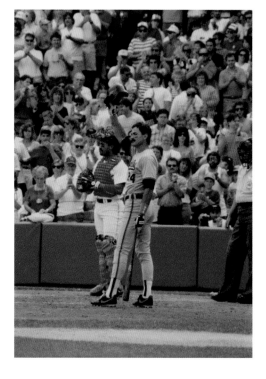

My final year of my big-league career in 1991 was with the Orioles. I never wanted to leave the Red Sox and was touched by the standing ovations every time I came to bat in my return to Fenway. (Dwight Evans Collection)

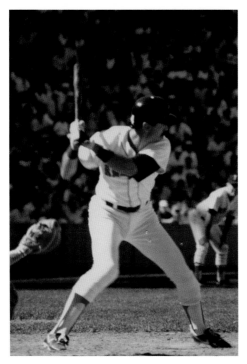

Taking my cuts at Fenway in 1988
during our drive for a division title.
(Dwight Evans Collection)

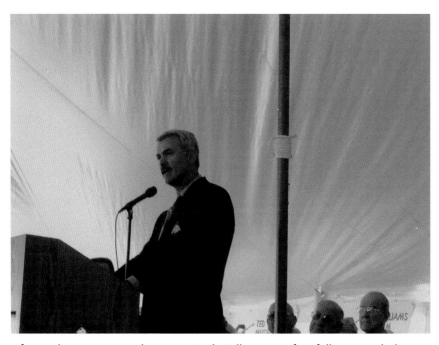

After a disastrous introduction to Ted Williams my first full year with the
Red Sox, it was sweet redemption to be inducted into his Ted Williams
Museum and Hitters Hall of Fame in 2002. (Dwight Evans Collection)

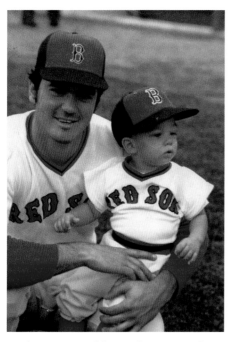

With one-year-old Timothy at a Red Sox Father–Son Game in 1974. (Dwight Evans Collection)

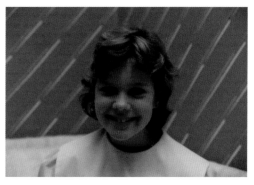

My daughter, Kirstin, at nine years old. While she was mercifully healthy, it wasn't easy for her because of all the time and care we had to give her brothers their entire lives. (Dwight Evans Collection)

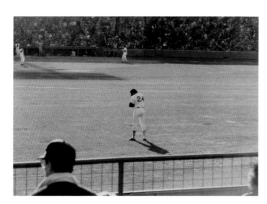

A moment of reflection between innings of a game in right field in 1985. Baseball had become a time-out and mental-free period from all my real-life problems. (Erik Sherman Collection)

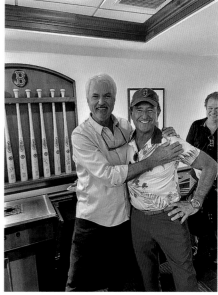

With Fred Lynn up in the Fenway Park Legends Suite in 2023. Freddie was a sensational centerfielder and we worked well patrolling the Red Sox outfield together for six full seasons. (Natalie Lynn)

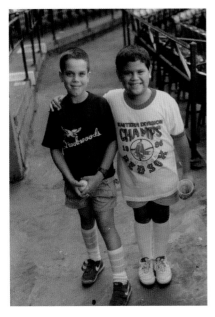

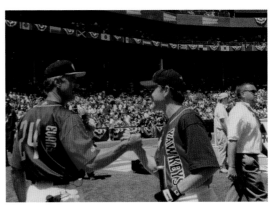

With actor Matt Damon at Fenway Park during All-Star Weekend in 1999. (Dwight Evans Collection)

Justin (on left) with the current Red Sox assistant general manager Eddie Romero. (Dwight Evans Collection)

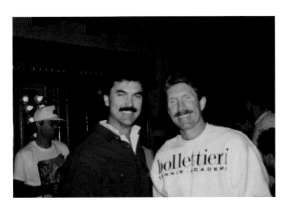

With Phillies legend Mike Schmidt during a Nike-sponsored trip to Arizona. During the decade of the 1980s, Schmidt hit the most home runs in the National League, and I had the most in American League. (Dwight Evans Collection)

Leaping in the air to grab a deep drive hit by Mike Davis in a game against the Oakland A's at Fenway as the home crowd looks on. I always understood and appreciated the passion of the Red Sox fans. (AP Photo/Peter Southwick)

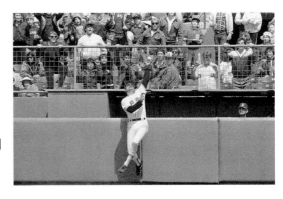

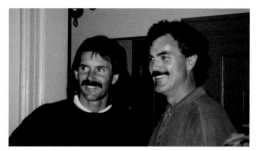

With Dennis Eckersley—a terrific pitcher, teammate, and friend.

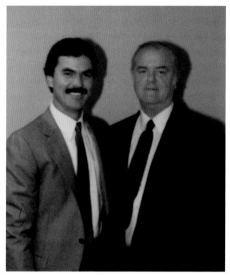

With my father, Duff. Because of his work, we moved numerous times when I was a child between Hawaii and Southern California. I was always the new kid on the block, which wasn't easy for me. (Dwight Evans Collection)

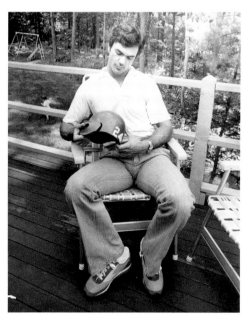

Holding my shattered helmet after taking a fastball behind my left ear in August 1978. I suffered a severe concussion and dealt with dizziness from vertigo for the next three years. (Courtesy: U.P.I)

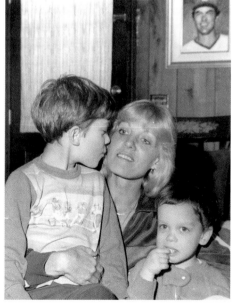

My wife, Susan, and the boys. While I was often away playing baseball, Susan had to handle everything that was being thrown at our family. (Dwight Evans collection)

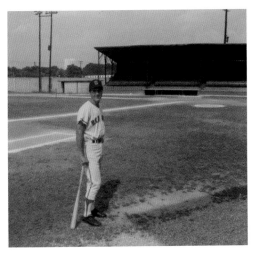

Playing A-Ball for the Greenville Red Sox in 1970. We won the Western Carolinas League title that year. (Dwight Evans collection)

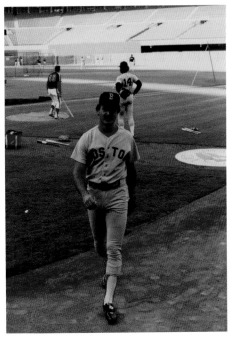

Pregame warm-ups prior to a 1986 ALCS game against the California Angels. (Dwight Evans Collection)

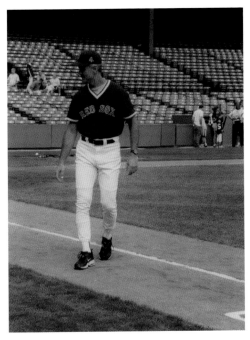

As a Red Sox coach in 2002. (Dwight Evans Collection)

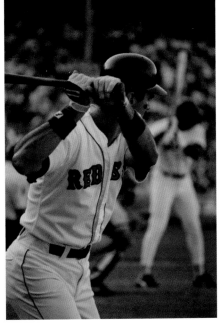

Waiting for my at-bat behind Don Baylor in 1986. (Dwight Evans Collection)

Susan and me with '86 Red Sox teammate and lifelong friend Don Baylor and his wife, Becky. (Dwight Evans Collection)

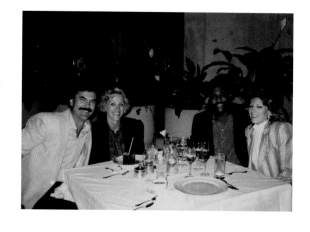

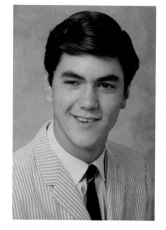

My senior picture from Chatsworth High School. In my senior year, I had a 6–0 pitching record to go along with a .552 batting average and was named the MVP of the West [San Fernando] Valley League. (Dwight Evans Collection)

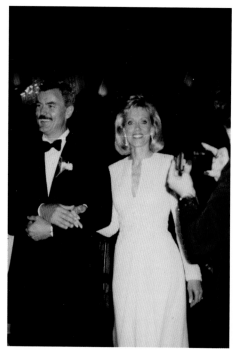

With Susan, the love of my life and wife of 53 years, at Kirstin's wedding. (Dwight Evans Collection)

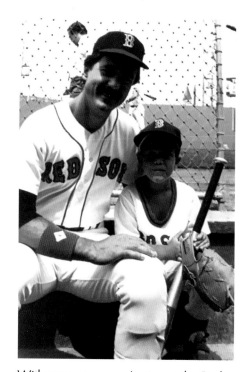

With youngest son, Justin, at the Red Sox Father-Son Game in 1984. (Dwight Evans Collection)

going. With my family now settled in the house we bought in Lynnfield, and with a degree of normalcy and structure in our lives, I was beginning to worry about logistics. *Would I have to live somewhere else away from my family?* It was a tough time.

When we went out to Anaheim earlier that month, Rick Miller, my former teammate who was now with the Angels, told me straight out that their owner, Gene Autry, thought he was going to be able to trade for me. It would have been interesting to play for the Angels because I was born in Santa Monica, moved away to Hawaii, and then from age 10 grew up in the San Fernando Valley. In a sense, it would have been like coming home. For as nice as that might sound, though, it may not have been a positive development in my life. I always thought that being in Boston was healthy for me. I know guys that went back to play in Southern California—like Lynn and Burleson—and they were constantly being asked by friends and family for tickets. It's a pain in the rear end to be dealing with stuff like that. I love my family, but sometimes when you're playing you don't have enough space for anything else except the game.

With trade rumors in the papers and on the airwaves, Susan decided to pull the sports section from our *Boston Globe*, telling me, "You don't need to see this," because she didn't want me to know what was being written about me or anybody else on the club. She only would tell me who the opposing pitcher was going to be that day. I also stopped listening to the car radio on the way to the ballpark. Whether something positive or negative was written or said about me didn't matter—I didn't need to hear it or see it in print. The strategy worked, and I started relaxing more both at the ballpark and at home.

Most importantly, the club surged out of the gates the first half of the season. As the All-Star break began on July 10, we were the class of major league baseball with an astounding 57–26 record.

We were in first place with a nine-game lead over second place Milwaukee, with an 11½-game edge over the Yankees and a 13-game advantage over the Orioles. We were running away with the division.

I wouldn't get much rest during the break—but for a *very good* reason. I had been named to my first All-Star team as a reserve outfielder. I would join teammates Burleson, Fisk, Lynn, Remy, Rice, and Yaz in San Diego. It was such a great feeling when I entered the game in right field in the fifth inning—replacing Richie Zisk—and looking out toward left field and seeing Rice, and then center field and seeing Lynn. It was an All–Red Sox outfield at the All-Star Game—a pretty special moment.

In the top of the eighth with two outs and nobody on base in a 3–3 game, I came up to bat against future Hall of Famer Bruce Sutter. I recalled Tim McCarver once telling me, "If you ever face Sutter, when he throws his forkball, the one you've got to hit is the one that starts up in the strike zone. If it comes in waist-high, lay off that one—it's going to drop off the table." Ironically, in this game, Sutter started me off with a forkball waist-high and, thinking it looked like a great pitch to hit (and not heeding McCarver's advice), I swung and missed just as the bottom dropped out of it. I had just seen how remarkable Sutter's forkball was firsthand. I managed to lay off the next three pitches—all out of the strike zone—to work the count to 3-1. Sutter then came back with two forkballs starting belt-high and, again, I couldn't lay off either of them before they dropped—and he struck me out to end the inning. All I could think was, *Ugh… McCarver was right.* But it truly was no sin striking out against Sutter. Rice, who was amidst one of the greatest seasons by any player in Major League history, fell victim to Sutter's forkball just before me, striking out in the same manner. There's a reason Sutter has a plaque in Cooperstown.

The National League would win the game 7–3, continuing its dominance over the American League in All-Star Games during that period with its seventh straight victory.

After dropping our first two games following the All-Star break, we went on a five game winning streak, reaching the apex of our season with a 62–28 record on July 19. Most significant was how we had built a 14-game lead over the defending world champion Yankees—their low point of the season. Our lineup was so potent that Hobson and I—often the eighth and ninth hitters—had almost as many home runs between us as the Cardinals, Cubs, or Padres. Throughout baseball history, you had lineups that included Ruth and Gehrig with the Yankees and Bobby Bonds, Mays, and McCovey with the Giants, but from one through nine, we had as strong a line-up as I had ever seen.

Meanwhile, in the Bronx, things were going from bad to worse to bizarre. On July 24, George Steinbrenner fired Billy Martin for derogatory comments the Yankees' manager made about him and Reggie Jackson. And then, less than a week later, during their Old Timers' Day ceremonies, they had Bob Sheppard, their public address announcer, announce that Martin would return as manager in 1980. It was like a soap opera over there. From our standpoint, the whole saga made for interesting reading, but we honestly didn't care. I figured it was time for Martin to go, anyway. He had a way of being successful with a club for two or three years, instilling a fear factor with certain players and getting away with it for a while. But then, in every case—with the Twins, Tigers, Rangers, and now with the Yankees—he would lose control of his team and get fired.

As for Steinbrenner, he was portrayed in the media as a real blowhard who wanted the spotlight to be more on himself than his players. And that's what I naturally thought by reading about him. But I'll never forget playing right field in Yankee Stadium

later in my career when I raced for a ball by the line and, while
leaping high up the wall to try to catch it, a fan threw a beer right
in my face. As a result, I lost the ball and didn't catch it. Following
the game, I was in the trainer's room getting some ice when the
phone rang and the clubby handed it over to me. "Hello Dewey,
it's George Steinbrenner," the voice on the line said. "Are you okay?
I want to apologize for our fans, and I just wanted you to know
that we got ahold of the guy that threw the beer at you and he'll
never be allowed back in Yankee Stadium again." It was a real
classy thing of George to do. After that, I had a whole different
perspective of him. And in the years that followed, I would hear
numerous stories of charity about Steinbrenner that would go
unreported—generosity that only those closest to him knew anything about. He once said, "If you do something good for some
other person and more than two people know about it, then you
didn't do it for the right reason." There's no doubt that George
could be very hard on his players and managers, but because he
was paying them a lot of money to produce, he understandably
expected strong results.

Now, Bob Lemon, an even-keeled, gentle man whose managing
style was the exact opposite from that of the fiery Martin, took
over the Yankees and vowed to simply fill out the lineup card
every day and just let the Yankees play. A newspaper strike in
New York, which would begin on August 10, would alleviate a
great deal of pressure the Yankee players were receiving for their
disappointing season to that point. And a Yankee team that had
its share of injuries started to get healthy again. All these factors
contributed to the Yankees playing better ball as the season moved
on into August.

As for us, we suddenly became the walking wounded. Injuries
are a part of the game, but what happened to us in mid-July and
early August was almost unprecedented. Burleson badly injured

his ankle sliding into second base; Fisk cracked his ribs; Remy cracked a bone in his wrist; Lynn was limping around with a sore back; Campbell developed arm stiffness and was never the same; Yaz was dealing with a bad back; Scott broke his middle finger; and Hobson had bone chips in his throwing elbow, which led to him making 43 errors that season.

Hobson was one of the toughest guys I ever played with. A lot of his injuries came from football—he had been a backup quarterback for the University of Alabama Crimson Tide under Coach Bear Bryant from 1969 through 1972. He told me he did a lot of damage to his right arm there, and that it was permanently bent—keeping him from fully extending it when making throws. But it never stopped him from playing. He was a determined, gritty player who was never going to use legitimate arm issues as an excuse for his throwing errors. But the bone chips had become so severe that Butch's backup, Jack Brohamer, would begin to see significant playing time.

Despite the injuries, on August 28 we still owned the best record in the majors with an 82–47 mark and a 7½-game lead over the surging Yankees. I was enjoying a big night against the Seattle Mariners at Fenway, collecting two doubles, a walk, and two RBIs. But then, in the bottom of the seventh, Mariners pitcher Mike Parrott seriously beaned me in the head right behind my left ear, shattering my helmet. I had to be carried off the field and taken to the hospital with a severe concussion. The dizziness from the vertigo I suffered from it was horrible. If I turned my head, things started spinning and I would get sick. If I walked off a curb and things started spinning, I would fall down. If I rolled over in bed, I would get nauseous. I had legitimate concerns about how it would affect my career.

Parrott was deeply distraught by the severity of the injury his beaning caused me. He was the first one on the field to run over and check on me. Parrott had some nasty stuff but was never the same pitcher after that, pitching his last major league game three years later at just 26 years old. His reaction to injuring me says a lot about the man.

Just five days later, I was back at the plate as a pinch-hitter. If that kind of serious concussion happened today, I would have been out for weeks, not days. In that at-bat, I managed to single in the ninth inning of a 4–3 loss to the A's at Fenway. Despite that promising first at-bat, I was really trash after the beaning. I was so afraid of getting hit in the head again—the extreme pain and vertigo from the beaning now embedded in my mind.

I was back out in right field the next night and anytime I put my head up, the vertigo set in. So, I began to just raise my eyes and keep my head still when catching fly balls. The vertigo really took a toll on me defensively that last month of the season, with four of the six errors I made all year coming just in September. I dealt with this problem for three years, but the symptoms were at their worst that first year.

At the end of play on September 6, we held a four-game lead over the second place Yankees and were set to host them for a crucial four-game series at Fenway. Our sizable lead hadn't been reduced the way it was because we had played terrible baseball— quite the contrary. Despite all the injuries, we still went 19–10 in August and were 2–4 in September (a .666 winning percentage over the period). It was just the Yankees were even hotter over that stretch, catching fire at the perfect time.

The weekend in New England that began on September 7 would be nothing short of a complete disaster and was dubbed "the Boston Massacre" by the local media. Torrez lasted just one-plus inning in the first game and the Yankees would go on to collect 21 hits on their way to a 15–3 romp. In the second game, rookie right-hander Jim Wright would only survive 1⅓ innings and the Yankees again won big 13–2. But it wasn't just the pitching that did us in. We committed seven errors, with Fisk and I committing two each. I continued to struggle mightily from my vertigo. With Eck going in the third game—even if it was against Ron Guidry, who was having a Cy Young season—it was our best chance to stop the bleeding. And it started off well enough, with both pitchers putting up zeros through three innings. But then the Yankees broke out and scored seven runs in the fourth and Eck's day was over. Guidry went the distance with a 7–0 shutout to improve his record to an astounding 21–2.

With our lead cut to just one game, Zim decided to give the ball to another rookie—left-hander Bobby Sprowl. In what was clearly one of our biggest games of the year, the players all wanted Zim to go with Bill Lee, who had pitched well out of the bullpen in the second game of the series—yielding just one earned run over seven innings—and certainly had the experience, confidence, and talent to get the job done. By contrast, Sprowl had exactly *one game* of major league experience. The Spaceman, who lived for these games, seemed like the logical choice. But Zim ignored the pleas of the players to go with Lee and left himself open to some major second-guessing by starting the rookie.

Sprowl wouldn't last the first inning—the moment just too big for the kid—as he walked four of the first six Yankees he faced, and New York took a 3–0 lead after one frame. Sprowl never recovered from the stress of that outing and would experience difficulties pitching hitters inside during spring training games for us the next year before being traded to Houston. He would only pitch another 33⅓ innings the rest of his brief big-league career.

It was only after the Yankees held a 7–3 lead with two outs in the top of the seventh that Zim would bring Lee into the game. Naturally, Spaceman pitched 2⅓ innings of shutout ball. For as well as he pitched against the Yankees, it would remarkably be Lee's last appearance in a Red Sox uniform.

The Yankees held on to win 7–4, completing a four-game sweep in which they outscored us 42–9 to move into a first-place tie. Our once 14-game lead over New York had evaporated with our ninth loss in 10 games.

Zimmer's handling of Lee put our quest for a division title in jeopardy. Zim positively hated him. Lee was 10–3 with an ERA of 2.94 on July 15, but losing seven straight games gave Zim the perfect excuse to remove Lee from the rotation. Zim never considered the fact that in five of those seven losses, Lee didn't give up more than three earned runs. Instead, Zim saw an opportunity to punish Lee for his quirky behavior and took advantage of it. August 19 would be Lee's last start of the season. There's no question in my mind that Lee would have won three or four more games down the stretch. And that's being conservative.

But Zim's hatred of Lee ran so deep that he put the best interests of the team after his personal feelings. The irony is that Zim was Lee's father's favorite player. Zim was a third baseman, just like Lee's dad, and they both had suffered severe beanings. Lee's father once asked his son, "How can you not get along with Zimmer?" Bill replied, "Dad, do we get along?" And he said, "You've got a point there."

With Lee and Zim, it was a conflict of personalities that got uglier after Bill mocked Zim publicly in '77, calling him a "gerbil." I love Bill, but some people thought he was goofy—and at times he was. He made public how he put marijuana on his pancakes and had the famous photo of himself in *Sports Illustrated* with his space suit on. He embraced being called Spaceman. And he did some funky things between starts that were not traditional, like kicking and throwing footballs to himself after infield practice at Fenway. He had fun. It didn't bother me at all because that's how he got his work in. But apparently his antics bothered some in the baseball establishment—including Zim. But when Lee got on the mound, he was all business, pitching to contact—a lost art. You knew with Lee out there you had a great chance to win.

Lee would be traded to the Montreal Expos after the season for Stan Papi, a journeyman utility infielder with limited big-league experience. Lee would win 16 games for the Expos the next season, quickly establishing himself as the ace of their staff. He would be missed.

––––––––––––––

Despite the four-game debacle against New York, there were still three weeks of baseball to be played. But after beating Baltimore in our first game after the Yankees series, we dropped our next five to fall 3½ games out of first place. But then, at last, we were able to stabilize matters and right the ship. We would finish the final two weeks of the regular season by winning 11 of our last 13 games, including an eight-game winning streak at the end. In the middle of our season-ending surge, the decision was made to move Rice to right field, as my vertigo persisted, relegating me to the bench in a pinch-hitting role. It was deeply distressing that for the second straight season, a serious injury curtailed what would have been an even more standout year for me personally. As it was, my twenty-four home runs were second on the club and the most of my career to that point.

The division race would come down to the final day of the season as the Yankees held a one-game lead over us. With Luis Tiant's two-hit shutout over Toronto at a delirious Fenway, we needed the Cleveland Indians—a 90-loss team—to find a way to beat the Yankees. Remarkably, they did just that, pounding Catfish Hunter early and often on their way to a 9–2 victory. Our

victory and the Yankees' loss gave us identical records of 99–63—
forcing a memorable one-game playoff at Fenway on October 2
to decide the division championship.

The general feeling on our side that bright Monday afternoon
was that losing a 14-game lead over the Yankees could be forgotten
with a single win in our own ballpark. We had gallantly battled
back from the brink to make this one-game playoff possible and,
as our eight-game winning streak heading into it attested, we
were not the chokers some in the media were portraying us as.

Torrez, who lived for the big game as evidenced by his two
complete game victories over the Dodgers in the '77 World Series,
would start for us against Guidry, who was seeking his 25th win of
the season. Just a little over two years before, Guidry had seriously
contemplated quitting baseball instead of reporting to Triple-A
Syracuse—miserable over how Billy Martin demoted him and
wanted the Yankees to trade him—before his wife talked him out
of it. At the time, he threw hard, but his slider was flat and very
hittable; and all his pitches came in at the same speed. But then
Sparky Lyle got a hold of him, taught him how to throw a hard
slider, and the rest is history. When you think about the worst
trades the Red Sox ever made, trading Lyle to the Yankees for
Danny Cater in 1972 must be at the top of the list. Not only did
the Red Sox trade a dominant reliever in Lyle who would win
the Cy Young Award in '77, but also a guy who would fix Guidry
and make him a dominant starting pitcher who would win the
Cy Young Award in '78.

The game started off as well as we could have hoped. For as
great as Guidry was that season, he was pitching on just three
days' rest and, as a result, might not have been as strong as usual.
Yaz led off the bottom of the second and got around well on a
Guidry fastball, ripping a home run inside the right-field foul
pole to give us a 1-0 lead. By this point, Yaz was 39 years old with

graying sideburns and a bad back, but he was still the anchor of our lineup. Carl was, indisputably, our revered leader, and was obsessed with winning a championship. It only made sense that he was the one that got things rolling for us.

Torrez was dealing on the mound, shutting out the Yankees through six frames. While he held the Yankees in check, we increased our lead to 2–0 in the bottom of the sixth when Burleson led off with a double and then was driven home by a one-out single by Rice. After Guidry issued Fisk a two-out intentional walk to put runners on first and second, Lynn came up to the plate. Lynn typically went the other way against the hard-throwing southpaw, but this time he hooked one into the right field corner in the area we called "Death Alley." Lou Piniella, who was playing right field instead of Reggie Jackson that day, ran toward the corner and snagged it for the out. If he doesn't get there in time, it's at least a double, we're up 4–0, Guidry is likely out of the game, we get into their middle-relief corps, and it's over. It was odd that Piniella was positioned where he was—close to the right field line playing Lynn to pull. Years later, Freddie asked Piniella about his positioning on that play. The astute Piniella told him, "Guidry was throwing a lot of innings. I didn't think he had his best stuff, so I moved over a little bit." It's that kind of thinking that the analytics can't teach you. Lou went by what he saw in Guidry, played his position accordingly, and saved two runs. It's not a play that's often talked about, but it may have been a game-saver for the Yankees.

The Yankees would mount their first serious threat in the top of the seventh. With one out, Torrez gave up singles to Chris Chambliss and Roy White. But after retiring pinch-hitter Jim Spencer on a harmless flyball to left field, it seemed like he was out of trouble. Bucky Dent, the Yankees' light-hitting shortstop who had hit just four home runs that season, came up to bat. The Yankees, who had just used Spencer to bat for second baseman Brian Doyle, had to allow Dent to hit because they ran out of infielders. All season long, they would pinch hit for Dent in this situation, but they couldn't do so here. With Willie Randolph injured and Doyle now out of the game, they only had Fred Stanley remaining on the bench to replace Doyle. So, it was up to Dent to keep their inning alive.

After taking the first pitch for a ball, Dent fouled the next one hard off his instep and fell to the ground in agony. There was a long delay while the Yankees' trainer, Gene Monahan, attended to Bucky. Aside from receiving medical attention, Bucky was given a new bat from Mickey Rivers. A lot has been said about whether there was something funny about that bat, but I have no idea if it was doctored. What I did know was that when Torrez threw a slider, it came from a different angle—more over the top—than his fastball. And that's something an opposing team could potentially pick up on. Anyway, no one was thinking Dent had much of a chance to hit a home run—especially after having just injured his foot.

But once play resumed, Torrez threw a slider down the middle and Dent hit it pretty well and high toward the Green Monster. At first, it looked like Yaz had a beat on it, but it kept carrying. As the flight of the ball began to descend, it scraped against the back of the wall and into the netting for a three-run homer to give the Yankees a 3–2 lead. It deflated us. And the ballpark, filled with so much electricity all game long, suddenly fell eerily silent and into a state of disbelief as Dent rounded the bases.

After walking the next batter (Rivers), Torrez's day was done. He really had pitched masterfully, but the one mistake pitch to Dent would be all most people would remember about his performance. Bob Stanley entered the game and, after Rivers stole second, Thurman Munson doubled to center field to increase the Yankees' lead to 4-2.

New York would increase their lead further in the top of the eighth when Jackson would hit a solo home run off Stanley into the center-field bleachers to give them a 5–2 lead.

But we battled back in our half of the eighth off Rich Gossage, who came in the previous inning to relieve Guidry. Yaz ripped a one-out RBI single to drive in Remy and then, two batters later, Lynn drove home Yaz to cut the deficit to 5–4. But with one out and Fisk and Lynn on base, we couldn't do any further damage against Gossage—it was a missed opportunity for sure.

The score would remain 5–4 into the bottom of the ninth. Zim called me over in the dugout to pinch hit for third baseman Frank Duffy, who had entered the game to replace Jack Brohamer. There was no speech about just getting on base from Zim—he wanted me to go deep against Gossage. "Take him out of here," he told me.

As I walked out to the batter's box, much of the crowd stood and started chanting "Dew-ey! Dew-ey! Dew-ey!" I wanted to come through in the worst way in one of the biggest at-bats of my career, but I was wary about being too anxious. Gossage could be wild. He was one of the most intimidating pitchers I ever faced. He threw as hard as Nolan Ryan did, but his arm angle came from over the hole at shortstop between third and shortstop. I took Gossage's first pitch low and away for a ball. The next pitch was what I was looking for—a fastball right over the plate, the kind of pitch I could drive out of the ballpark. I put a good swing on it but just got a hair under it, sending a fly ball to left field for the first out of the inning. Another eighth of an inch and I would have squared it up and sent it a long way to possibly tie the game, but it wasn't to be.

But we weren't dead yet. Gossage, showing signs of wildness, threw three straight balls to Burleson before walking him on a 3-1 count to put the tying run on first. Remy was up next and, on an 0-2 count, drilled a line drive to right field. Piniella, looking right up into the sun, didn't see the ball, but put his arms out to his sides and, at the last possible moment, caught the ball in his glove on one hop before it got by him. By putting his arms up, he froze Burleson long enough so his perfect throw to third base kept the Rooster at second. By not panicking, and by not waving his arms, Burleson couldn't tell that Piniella lost the ball. To this day, I don't know how he did what he was able to do on that play. If the ball got by Piniella, with Remy's speed, it could have been a division-winning, inside-the-park home run. Piniella was not a great outfielder, but his instincts were off the charts. It was simply a remarkable, game-saving play. With his catch of Lynn's flyball earlier in the game, Piniella saved at least three runs that afternoon with his defense and instincts.

What Piniella's play on Remy's single also did was keep the tying run on second, so a long flyball was not going to tie the game. And that was critical with Rice coming to bat next. And sure enough, with Gossage throwing Rice nothing but heat, Jimmy hammered one deep to right—deep enough to move Burleson to third with a long sacrifice fly. Had the Rooster been able to reach third on Remy's single, Rice's drive would have tied the game. Jimmy didn't miss hitting a home run by much on that pitch, but the ball didn't carry well at Fenway late in the season. The air is cooler, and the wind blows differently during the fall. You really had to hit a bomb to get one to leave the ballpark.

So now, with runners on first and third and two outs, that brought up Yaz with the game and our season on the line. He was definitely the right person up at the right time. I liked the matchup. After taking the first pitch for a ball, Yaz got the fastball he was looking for, but he was slightly late on it, popping it up near third where Nettles caught it to end the game and clinch the division title for the Yankees.

For baseball fans, the game was a classic. For us, it was a devastating end to a season that for months held so much promise. Despite an overwhelming number of injuries, we still won 99 games. I've often wondered how winning that many games—the second-most in baseball in '78—could be a big disappointment. Our team is still ridiculed by a lot of people in Boston because of the big lead we let slip away. But no one talks about how well the Yankees played to come back and overtake us. And it's seldom brought up how we won eight straight games at the end of the season to force the one-game playoff.

Our '78 club may have been the most talented I ever played on. As such, there was a very different mindset after losing this one-game playoff compared to when we lost Game Seven of the 1975 World Series. In '75, we were a team on the rise with a mix of young players like Lynn, Rice, Burleson, myself, and others. So, after we lost Game 7 to the Big Red Machine on a bloop single by Joe Morgan, there was disappointment, but we knew there was so much upside potential that we would have multiple chances to win the World Series in the years ahead. But '78 was different. It wasn't about our potential. We already knew who we were and how good we were. We knew we could win eight in a row down the stretch to force the playoff game. We hated this loss because we knew we were better than the Yankees. And despite the season we had, we couldn't even get into the playoffs. So, it was a different kind of hurt—a far more devastating hurt. Perhaps worst of all, we didn't know how much longer we would all be together.

Well, a month later we found out. The Yankees would rip our hearts out again by signing free agent Luis Tiant.

Was this the beginning of the end of the Red Sox dynasty that never was?

Only time would tell.

CHAPTER 12

SINKING SHIP

IT COULD HAVE BEEN CATASTROPHIC.

During the off-season prior to the 1979 campaign, Yaz invited me to his home in Highland Beach on the east coast of Florida for 10 days of fishing. Each morning, we went out on his boat at 6:00 AM. Those were bonding times.

But on this one day, our lives were suddenly in danger. There was a strong Gulf Stream current in the Atlantic Ocean about three miles out. The current is like a wall of water that ranges from two feet to as high as six feet, so you would have to build up some speed with your boat to get over it. So, while we were fishing for mahi-mahi, we noticed stuff floating around us like boards and other pieces from wrecks—a sign of rough waters, but not unusual. But 20 minutes later, we were stunned to see the mahi-mahis we had caught swimming around us in the boat. We were taking on water!

The front of our boat was now out of the water and the back was pretty much full of water. The bilge pump, used to pump water out of the boat, had gone out. Worse yet, our twin engines had failed and were shut off. So, while I was desperately trying to bail the water out of the boat (without pails), Yaz was trying to start up the engines again. In doing so, Yaz discovered that one of the power cables to the batteries connected to the two engines was singed off because there was water in it.

At this point, I was praying. *What do we do now?* Trying to remain as composed as possible, I said, "Carl, I'm going to take this cable and try to hook it up to the part where it's singed off. When I do that, try to start the engine back up." *It worked!*

For the next three hours, we slowly navigated the boat back to shore with the entire front end out of the water. It wasn't pretty, but we were just so thankful to get back safely. It was a life-flashing moment in time.

The boating incident would prove to be a metaphor for our 1979 season, as the club also began taking on water before sinking to a generational low record in 1983.

Luis Tiant's departure had not only taken away one of our best starting pitchers, but also strengthened a division rival's rotation. And because he exited via free agency, we received nothing in return. There was no doubt Luis was nearing the end of his career, but he could still pitch. And what he meant to us as a leader and as a fan favorite in the eight years he pitched for the Red Sox cannot be overstated. The image of seeing him finish his warm-up pitches, wiping his forehead with a towel, throwing it down as if to say, *Let's Go!*, and then being greeted with a standing ovation the moment that bullpen latch opened, will remain in my memory for as long as I live. I've never seen anything like it since. And now that key element of our club was gone for good.

Three weeks later, Lee was traded to the Expos for Stan Papi, who would hit .188 in '79 and be gone the following year. Spaceman, meanwhile, had his best year in four seasons, winning 16 games in 33 starts for Montreal.

Losing them both left us woefully short on starting pitching—wasting the efforts of another powerful batting lineup that again produced big numbers.

But the purge wouldn't stop there. A little more than two years after the departures of Tiant and Lee, we lost Burleson, Lynn, Scott, Hobson, and Fisk via trade or free agency. In Fisk's case, we lost a New England guy—it was previously inconceivable that he would ever play for any club other than the Red Sox. There was no replacing him. But in January '81, Carlton was declared a free agent because co-owner and general manager Haywood Sullivan failed to send out his contract in time. Carlton would sign with the Chicago White Sox that March. On his way out, I remember him saying of the Red Sox, "The direction is hopeless."

It was hard losing a big part of the core of that immensely talented 1977–78 team. I didn't think things were hopeless, as Fisk said, but I did believe the club was seriously damaged. The question of concern I had was, *Who's running the ball club?* We now had three owners in Sullivan, Jean Yawkey, and Buddy LeRoux and it seemed little was running smoothly, leading to some major gaffes including the Fisk fiasco.

But at least there was one positive amid this tumultuous period. I truly hit my stride as a hitter, making adjustments at the plate that would pay major dividends for the rest of my career. In July of 1980, I was hitting just .188 and was being platooned with Jimmy Dwyer. The beaning that I suffered in '78 had a long-term effect on me in several ways. Although much of my vertigo was now gone, I had gotten into some bad habits.

Enter Red Sox coach Walt Hriniak, a guru on hitting with a unique set of batting theories. Walt gave me an ultimatum, exclaiming, "If we work together, you've got to stay with me, and you need to see this through. You can't can it after a week—you've got to stay with it." I pledged that I would.

The first thing Walt impressed upon me was to stay balanced at the plate. By not being balanced, I was more vulnerable to getting hit by pitches. The second thing he stressed was head discipline.

That's why I still, to this day, tell hitters, *You've got to keep your head down where you're striking the ball. If your head pulls out, you're gone.* When I see hitters getting violent with their swing, their head usually flies out, so keeping it down to the ball is critical. And number three, Walt wanted me to get back to hitting line drives into the middle of the field—from right-center to left-center.

Zimmer was skeptical about Hriniak's approach to hitting. "I'll be doggone if I'd teach anybody to hit singles up the middle," he told me. But Zim was missing the point. Walt wanted me to drive the ball and said the home runs would come naturally—just more toward the middle of the field. The improvement in my hitting was almost immediate. I hit well over .300 the rest of the '80 season to finish at .266 with 18 home runs. I had made a complete, drastic change to my hitting approach at 28 years old.

With five games remaining in a 1980 campaign in which we would finish in fourth place and 19 games out (which followed a third-place finish in 1979), the Red Sox fired Zim, replacing him with interim manager Johnny Pesky for the remainder of the season. I loved Zim, but I felt a change could be a positive for the team with the right manager. As it turned out, the Red Sox couldn't have picked a better man for the job.

The hiring of Ralph Houk as our new manager for 1981 changed my career. I can't overstate how monumental it was for me. At the start of spring training, he called me into his office for a meeting. "I looked at your stats," he told me. "You led the team in on-base percentage hitting at the bottom of the order. I'm moving you up to the leadoff spot. You're going to get one more at-bat per game." Houk justified his moving me to the top of the order with the media, telling them, "The guy has power, and I don't mind leading him off and maybe starting with a 1–0 lead."

I couldn't wait for the spring training games to start. In our opening game in Winter Haven, for the first time in my career, I started looking for pitches in certain areas of the plate. In my first at-bat, I got the pitch I was looking for and hit a bomb to right center for a triple. From there, I never stopped hitting throughout spring training, leading the Red Sox in home runs. I continued to hit at a torrid pace into the first few weeks of the regular season and Houk moved me to third in the lineup before ultimately instilling me into the two spot later in the year.

But for as well as the season was progressing for me, it was very nearly derailed under the most tragic of circumstances. Following our April 29 game in Texas, Yaz and I were *very fortunate* to have survived a fatal three-car accident that killed six young people and injured two others.

Carl and I had a friend named Richard Thiessen who would fly in and watch some of our games, so we made plans to meet him for dinner in Dallas. But instead of waiting for the team bus to take us from Arlington into Dallas, we jumped in a cab. Our taxi was driving in the middle eastbound lane of Interstate 30 between Dallas and Fort Worth when a man—in an attempted act of suicide—drove his speeding car 80 mph the wrong way and sent it head-on into a car with seven young passengers returning from the game just ahead of us in the fast lane. I remember seeing his lights coming right at us and the car carrying all those people spinning before getting pummeled. Everything just exploded. Bodies, tires, and car parts were flying everywhere over and around us. Our taxi driver jammed on his brakes hard, but we still hit the car that lost those people, totaling the front end of our cab. It was mystifying to me how nothing came through our windshield. And it was nothing short of a miracle that nothing happened to us—not even a scratch. We got out of our taxi and ran toward the wreckage to see if we could help anybody. The driver and two of his passengers in the car in front of us were killed instantly. To this day, I still recall what it was like to stand over this beautiful 20-year-old girl—her stunning blue eyes wide open and lifeless, her body severely mangled. In my mind, I can still see her face.

Yaz and I eventually got back to our hotel late that evening and were very shaken up over what we had just witnessed. We talked about how we couldn't imagine the victims' parents getting the horrible phone calls that followed the accident. We later found out that three others involved in the crash died at the hospital, though the suicidal driver survived. The tragedy still bothers me today. It makes me think of my grandkids. I think of those innocent young people and how this one idiot decided to drive onto a highway to commit suicide and took out a carload of kids like he did. The visual of that night was life-changing. I get emotional just thinking about it.

—————————

Despite the mental toll the car accident took on me in the weeks afterward, by the end of play on June 11, I was leading the league in hitting with a .341 average and was right near the top in home runs and RBIs. In our June 11 game in Anaheim, despite going 0-for-4, I hit four bullets right at people. I couldn't wait to play the next day. But that next day never happened.

The only thing that could stop my hot streak in '81 was the start of a seven-week baseball strike that began on June 12. The Major League Baseball Players' Association (MLBPA) gave an ultimatum to the owners that if we didn't have a new contract in place, we were striking. Earlier that year, the owners had, without MLBPA approval, unilaterally implemented a compensation plan under which a team signing a free agent would give up a roster player and an amateur draft choice. We felt this plan undermined the value of free agency and we were never going to allow that to happen.

The long and bitter strike ended on July 31 with compromises on three major issues. One, teams losing a "premium" free agent could pick from a pool of players left unprotected from all the clubs rather than just the signing club. Two, the MLBPA agreed to restrict free agency to players with six or more years of major league service. Three, there was a raise in the minimum player salary. The fans were really frustrated with the players at that time, calling us greedy among other choice words. But what the fans didn't know—and even the players didn't realize until later in the year—was that the owners had taken out an insurance policy with Lloyd's of London—*before the strike*—to the tune of $44 million. While the players were losing salary every day the strike went on, the owners got their insurance money to cover much of their losses. Lloyd's of London, like all insurance entities, was like a gambling company. In this case, they believed there was no way that baseball was going to stop in America. But the owners wouldn't consider a compromise, much less serious negotiations, until their insurance money was nearly dried up. Once it got close to being exhausted, the strike was settled within a couple of days. The result of the strike was the cancellation of 712 games or 38 percent of the regular season. The relationship between the owners and players would never be the same.

My next game wouldn't come until I played in the All-Star Game on August 9 at Cleveland's Municipal Stadium—the Major League's first contest after the strike ended. In the fourth inning, I entered the game as a pinch-hitter for Reggie Jackson and drew a walk against Bob Knepper. Then, in the sixth inning, I got my first All-Star Game base hit—a line drive single to right field off Burt Hooton—and later came around to score on a Buddy Bell single to give the American League a 3–2 lead. But the National League would prevail once again, winning the game 5–4 on home runs by Dave Parker, Mike Schmidt, and two from the game's MVP, Gary Carter.

Because of the length of the strike, the owners decided to split the 1981 season into two halves. The first-place teams in each division from both halves would meet in a best-of-five divisional playoff series at the conclusion of the regular season. If a team won both halves in their division, it would face the second half runner-up instead. With this being the case, we were getting a fresh start after finishing the first half in fifth place.

Once we were back on the field, I could not quite get that feeling I had at the plate in the first half. But I still had the best season I ever had to that point in my career, hitting .296 and leading the American League in home runs, total bases, walks, and OPS (on-base plus slugging). I was awarded my first Silver Slugger Award, would win the first in a string of five straight Gold Glove Awards, and would finish third in the MVP voting. I say this humbly, but I really thought I should have won the MVP Award that season—and I wasn't alone. Even the actual MVP winner, Rollie Fingers, would tell reporters, "I really thought the guy in Boston could have won it." That made me feel good and showed what a class act Fingers was.

As a club, we played good baseball in the "second season," finishing in second place with a 29–23 record. Overall, if there would not have been a split-season, we would have finished with a 59–49 record and just 2½ games out of first place. As a result, there were reasons for future optimism. In fact, we were already beginning to see some of the ingredients for our next championship run in 1986 with the call-ups of pitcher Bruce Hurst and catcher Richie Gedman. They don't make better people than those two—both men were very caring and sensitive individuals who would overcome major challenges to become stars in the big leagues.

Gedman was signed by the Red Sox as a non-draftee amateur free agent, got called up from the minors at just 20 years old, was the runner-up in the Rookie of the Year voting in '81, was a two-time All-Star in '85 and '86, and would play 13 seasons in the majors. Richie proved everyone wrong at every level he played at, improving his catching skills to become a really solid receiver—all with the added pressure of taking over the role after Fisk's departure.

Hurst had fine control and a great breaking ball right from the outset of his career. But I said to the young Hurst when we were shagging fly balls in the outfield one time, "Bruce, you've got to come up with a change-up." Oh boy, did he get mad at me. "What are you?!" he asked. "Are you a *pitching coach* now?" I don't know if he listened to my advice or not, but Bruce did, in fact, come up with a forkball and it changed his career. He truly became a great pitcher after that. The forkball made his fast ball and breaking ball look even better. He mastered that pitch, throwing it in the strike zone as well as dropping it outside the strike zone almost whenever he wanted.

On any club with young, promising players, you need veterans with a championship pedigree to demonstrate to them how to play winning baseball. One such player we had on that club from 1980 through 1982 was Tony Perez, the backbone of the 1970s Big Red Machine. I will never forget an instance when I came up with a man on second base and nobody out. I hit a hellacious line drive right at the second baseman's knees. The shot handcuffed him, but he was able to hold on and make the catch. The runner had to hold at second. I come trotting into the dugout and all my teammates except for one were telling me things like, *Nice try, Dewey, Nice rip, Dewey.* The one who didn't was Tony Perez. Tony just sat on the bench with his arms crossed before asking me with that deep voice of his, "You think you did a good job?"

I said, "Well, I hit a line drive to the right side." Tony put up his index finger, started moving it from side to side, and looked me dead square in the face and said, "You didn't do the job. You didn't get the runner over." And I go, "You're right—I didn't get the job done." Tony taught me something that day and it rubbed off on the entire team.

We showed further improvement in '82, with more of the building blocks of the '86 team coming into play. Wade Boggs had a tremendous rookie year, hitting .349. Oil Can Boyd got his first taste of big-league life and would soon play an integral role on our pitching staff. And then there was second baseman Marty Barrett, who would turn out to be one of the smartest players I ever played with. He was a student of the game and a team player who always wanted to do better. Even as a rookie, he did things that usually you would only see a veteran do, like picking a pitcher apart to see if he was tipping his pitches. He was always doing things that were on edge, and he was always thinking. He would have made a terrific big-league manager had he had the opportunity.

I took to Marty right away because of how he respected the game and the veterans on the club. One time during his rookie year, Marty was in the middle of the line to get on the team bus when Yaz and I decided to have a little fun with him. "Back of the line, Rook!" we told him. So, Marty immediately starts to head to the back when Yaz laughs and grabs him by the arm and says, "No, no, no, you're okay." There was no arrogance to Marty and that element was very special in a young player who had just come up. You could tell he was very educated in every intricacy of the game both on and off the field.

We spent much of the first four months of the '82 season in first place and there was excitement back at Fenway. But all that enthusiasm took a back seat to a horrific scene—and act of heroism—at the ballpark on August 7, 1982. Before nets were put up at all the major league ballparks to protect the spectators, I would always cringe when a screaming line drive was hit into the stands. On this day, our shortstop Dave Stapleton hit a line drive foul that just smoked four-year-old Jonathan Keane seated a few rows behind our on-deck circle. Jimmy Rice looked out from the dugout, saw the severity of the situation, jumped into the stands, grabbed little Jonathan, and rushed him into our clubhouse for treatment before he was rushed to Boston's Children's Hospital. It was this great reaction by Jimmy that likely saved the boy's life.

We finished the '82 season with 89 wins and in third place, six games behind the division-winning Milwaukee Brewers. I played in all 162 games and put up the best numbers of my career to date with 32 home runs and 98 RBIs while leading the American League with a .402 on-base percentage. I would finish seventh in the MVP voting. But most importantly, the team was making strides and I felt our prospects were good for the following season. However, I was still deeply concerned with the direction and long-term stability of the club as the internal strife within ownership continued.

After Mr. Tom Yawkey died in 1976, the organization was run pretty much the same way under his widow, Mrs. Jean Yawkey. Under the Yawkeys, the Red Sox were a first-class operation. They went through some things where some players from other teams would say things like, "I'm not going to Boston. Yawkey is a racist." Much of that came from the fact that the Red Sox were the last major league team to have a Black player on the big-league roster. Pumpsie Green came a full 12 years after Jackie Robinson broke the color barrier with the Brooklyn Dodgers. But I didn't see any form of racism at all when I played under Mr. Yawkey. Of course, being white, maybe I was oblivious to it, but I can only go by what I observed. And what I saw was how Mr. Yawkey would come into the clubhouse and check in on *everybody*. There was a locker between Reggie Smith (an African American) and Yaz, and he would sit between them and talk to them both for 10 and 15 minutes at a time. I felt that it didn't matter what color you were; if you could play baseball and play it well, you could play for the Boston Red Sox.

But after Haywood Sullivan and Buddy LeRoux became partners with Jean Yawkey in 1981, everything changed. The way we would travel and the shortcuts were taking a toll on the players. For example, if we had a night game in Seattle, we would have to fly commercial the next morning at 7:30 AM, which is unheard of. You can't just wake up at 7:00 AM and get on a plane. We were hardly getting any sleep. The guys would come to me as one of the elder statesmen and complain. I was their clubhouse lawyer. But it was hard listening to all the complaints and not being able to do anything about it. It just didn't feel like the Boston Red Sox anymore.

In fact, I became so frustrated with the entire situation that I called a press conference two weeks before reporting to spring training in 1983 to demand a trade. And being a year or so away from free agency, I was prepared to go elsewhere. It wasn't so much about the money but about the way the club had been run the previous two seasons. I wanted to be on not just a competitive team, but also one that treated major league players—an elite group of individuals—with more respect. I watched one player after another not be tendered a contract by the December 20 deadline and become free agents. The Red Sox had become directionless.

I ended up staying with the Red Sox, hoping my behavior and all the noise I made would improve matters. I was looking forward to what I anticipated could be a great campaign and for all the well-deserved attention that would be paid to my dear friend Yaz in the final season of his storied career.

Since our last great season in 1978, Yaz was making the biggest headlines on the club by recording his 3,000th hit and 400th home run. In doing both, he became the first American League player to accomplish the feat. When his 23rd and final season came to a glorious end, at age 43, he would finish with 452 home runs and 3,419 hits.

Yaz's final season was a special time, fun to watch, and part of baseball history. Carl was not a big man in stature, measuring 5'11" and weighing 175 pounds throughout his career. How he got all he did out of his body still mystifies me in a lot of ways. He played through a lot of pain and taught Rice and me how to play—*and produce*—through injuries. It's not enough to just show up and play with pain—you've got to be able to play well to make an impact.

I recall during the 1977 All-Star Game, the American League manager Billy Martin put Carl in center field. Carl was really hobbling from an injury he was playing through but went out there anyway. That's a "gamer." I think that word was invented for Carl.

As we were closing out an unexpectantly disappointing 1983 season at 78–84—the Red Sox's worst record since 1966—and finished in sixth place, 20 games out, Yaz's farewell ceremony at Fenway Park was the only thing we had to look forward to.

Following a wonderful speech he gave on the field the day before the last game of the season, Yaz ran around the entire field, touching the outreaching hands of hundreds of fans standing along the front row of the lower box seats. It was a unique gesture by Yaz that I had never seen any athlete do before. Yaz didn't show emotion all the time, but he loved the fans, he loved New England, and he loved the Boston Red Sox. He understood and appreciated what we meant to the region.

In the clubhouse, away from everything he received on the field, our guys got together and presented him with a solid brass fishing rod as a retirement gift. It was beautiful. Yaz's sendoff ended an otherwise tough season on a high note. And it was truly the end of an era in Red Sox history.

CHAPTER 13

FAITH, DESPAIR, AND SPIRITUAL HOME RUNS

WHILE EVERY FACET OF THE GAME had come together for me as a ballplayer in the early '80s, my family life was bringing me to my knees. Much of what I faced during this period was far more distressing and intense than anything I ever faced on the playing field.

With Timothy already having suffered from NF for several years by the winter of '81–82, my youngest child, Justin—still a preschooler—out of nowhere began having massive, horrific migraines. He would hide under our couch because the pain was so bad. We took him in for a CAT scan at Brigham and Women's Hospital and received the devastating diagnosis—our little boy had an inoperable brain tumor, a symptom of NF. Our worst fears were realized. Both boys were now suffering from this horrific condition.

Dr. Israel Abrams told us, "When Justin starts to lose his vision, we're going to have to do radiation." Soon thereafter, Justin began losing his sight so we started the radiation process to burn the tumor. Dr. Abrams prepared us for the worst. "His vision won't come back," he said. But Justin was the happiest and most optimistic child in the world, and perhaps it was his positive attitude that served him well in the unlikeliest of recoveries. Halfway through the radiation process, the doctors performed some tests on him. Remarkably, Justin's condition was *improving*. After some more tests a few days later, his vision had improved some more. "I'm healed!" Justin exclaimed—if a bit prematurely—to the doctor. "That's nice," Dr. Abrams said to Justin. "Good boy." But then, after the final set of tests, Susan was at home when the phone rang with the results. Dr. Abrams laughed before saying, "It's all gone. It's all gone. His vision has been restored. He's fine." It was nothing short of a miracle.

However, it wasn't long before we had other grave concerns with Justin. The radiation had destroyed his pituitary glands, stunting his growth. We had to begin injecting Justin daily with the growth hormone Protropin for the next 12 years. I was so nervous the first time I gave him a shot. He had his thigh hanging out, wearing a pair of shorts, and as soon as I jammed the needle into his leg, I pulled it right back out as a reflex because he immediately started crying. I wanted to cry with him. But because I pulled it right out, I had to give him the shot all over again. Susan gave him the shots after that.

Another disturbing incident occurred shortly thereafter when we were doing chores around the house. Whenever I put something in Justin's hands, like a little split log to carry over to a pile, it just dropped straight to the ground. His debility continued until after I went to spring training in March of '82 when one morning he was getting ready for kindergarten when he realized he couldn't hold a pen in his right hand. In fact, Justin was having an issue with his entire right side, yet he still dragged himself up into the school bus. Susan immediately called the Red Sox medical director, Dr. Arthur Pappas, and told him what was happening. "Where is he now?" Dr. Pappas asked Susan. "I sent him to school," she said. "You're one tough broad," he answered. "Go get him out of school and come see me right away."

After numerous tests were performed on Justin, a tumor was found at the base of his brain, which had been affecting him physically and needed to come out right away. A very long and dangerous surgery at UMass Medical Center followed, one in which Justin almost died on the table. But with the expertise of some great surgeons under the leadership of Dr. Pappas, and after a lengthy recovery period which lasted for several months, Justin pulled through. I really cannot say enough about Dr. Pappas. He was such a caring individual who looked after all of us through a tough time. Some doctors see what they do as a job, while others, like Dr. Pappas, have a passion to help people. We were blessed to have him.

Still, both Susan and I were overwhelmed by the dire circumstances we were going through with our two very sick boys, and it was affecting us mentally and physically. Because of all the stress, Susan became borderline anorexic and chain-smoked three packs of cigarettes a day. She stood 5'8" and saw her weight drop close to 30 pounds over this period, to just 105 pounds. Her body was basically feeding off her organs. Susan would say she couldn't control anything in her life except her eating—or lack thereof. Neither one of us was happy with our lives. Instead, we just existed. At least I was able to drive to the ballpark, pull into the parking lot, and play a baseball game. It was like a timeout from real life—a mental free period that lasted six or seven hours. But I can't imagine what Susan was going through being alone half the time, handling everything that was being thrown at our family.

We were at a breaking point in our marriage. We were just always butting heads. We were around nice couples who served as strong examples for us—and we still had some good times together—but once I went away, she would be by herself. For me, it was frustrating to be away from the family. I felt like less of a man through those times when I couldn't be there to lend more support. And we didn't have the money then to bring someone in to help Susan out. With most players at that time, if you saved a little bit of money, you were doing well. But most guys still had to work in the off-season. I'm not saying money was the answer, but it would have helped.

We saw a therapist for a while until that ran its course. The one thing we had going for us was a mutual belief in commitment—through thick and thin, through tough times and good times. We had two very sick children. *What could we do?* I've often thought about what it would have been like if we had separated or even divorced. What kind of man would I have been? What kind of woman would she have been? What kind of people would we have been if we just gave up on our marriage because of the stress brought on by our boys' medical conditions? Every marriage has its ups and downs. And I know plenty of guys who left their marriages because they weren't happy. *For what?* The grass isn't always greener on the other side.

We tried to handle everything we possibly could as human beings. But it wasn't enough. We were hurting. But just as we were feeling helpless over our situation, a dramatic turning point occurred in our lives. I was wrapping up a long West Coast trip with the club in Oakland when three men of faith—two African Americans and a white person—drove all the way from Pittsburgh to our home in Lynnfield, Massachusetts, to see us. They started their trip with just $20 but were graciously given money by strangers along the way. The men had read an article about our personal strife and were on a mission to help us. They didn't have our address, so their first stop was Fenway Park to get it. They asked a Red Sox employee where we lived and were told he couldn't give out that kind of information. After one of the men ultimately told the employee, "God has sent us to see them," convinced of their righteousness and sincerity, he told them we lived in Lynnfield. From there, the three men stopped at a fire station in our town, asking a fireman for our address. The fireman said he couldn't give that out. One of the men said, "Well, the Lord has sent us." The fireman, sensing the reverence of the three pious men, finally acquiesced, and said, "Okay, Dwight lives at 3 Jordan Road." When they arrived at our front door, the men explained to Susan why they were there. She was clearly at a crossroads and had to make a split-second decision. She could turn them away or let them in and possibly change our lives. Susan just sort of stood there for a moment, unsure of what to do, when one of them said, "God sent us to you to tell you He loves you." That's when Susan opened her heart and let them in. It's likely at the very moment those men knocked on our door, I was reading the Bible—First Revelations 3:15 and 3:16—in my hotel room. The message of the two verses is that if you're going to live for God, live wholeheartedly or not at all—not "lukewarm." And that verse changed my life from that day forward.

After coming home from my road trip, I told Susan I had something to tell her. And she told me she had something to tell me. We hadn't spoken in 10 days and decided to have dinner together at the Union Oyster House in Boston. It's one of the oldest restaurants in Boston and we sat in the booth where John F. Kennedy dined. We shared our stories with one another about the messages we had received from God.

It was at that time when we had an awakening. We realized life couldn't go on as it had been going. We couldn't handle everything on our own. God had come into our lives, and we realized we could leave it all up to Him. God is the same yesterday, today, and tomorrow. God chooses to heal some and not others. I don't know why that is, but that will be a question that I will have until my time of passing on into heaven. Through our faith in God, suddenly all that burden that was on us kind of disappeared. And when Susan recommitted to Christ and I accepted Him for the first time, I realized how much more I loved her and how much more she loved me. Some people don't understand this, which is fine. But I really want the people who might not understand to know that our faith became the glue to our marriage and has kept us together for more than 50 years now.

While we were doing everything we could to make sure that Timothy and Justin were receiving all the medical care they needed, we also had to be sensitive to their emotional needs, as well. In Timothy's case, we would take him to a therapist and the four of us would sit together and address the embarrassment he felt over the teasing he received at school, as well as how to cope with his learning disabilities. Because his learning was all verbal, kids would tell him things that were just so wrong, yet he believed them because that was the only way he learned. Timothy got into a lot of fights defending himself over the teasing. Kids can be so cruel, and some called him "One Eye." That hurt all of us very deeply. The bullying was awful and didn't just take place at school. Even some of my teammates' kids would give him a hard time and he would sometimes hide under his seat at the ballpark so they wouldn't see him. The only time Tim felt comfortable and normal was when he was in the hospital, because all the other kids had a problem, too. No one was staring or pointing at him there. Timothy wanted so badly to be a baseball player like me, but he knew that was never going to happen. There were times when Timothy wanted to give up.

While Susan and I thought we were doing all we could for him, it apparently wasn't enough. The therapist had Susan and I meet separately with her, as well, to learn how to best work with Timothy to overcome his sadness and anxieties over his condition.

We always tried to keep his spirits up and tell him how proud we were of him. I always told Timothy, and later Justin, that they were my heroes when I took them in for their surgeries. And I meant it. They knew what was happening and they kept fighting with tremendous desire.

With Justin, his faith was strong and always in his heart from the time he was a very small child. One night at a church service, Justin, at just five years old, went up to someone there and told them, "I need to sing. I need to sing." And he got up on a stage with a microphone and belted out a rendition of "Jesus Loves Me." He sang his heart out—you could see the veins in his neck bulging out. It was just so awesome. During hospital visits for his treatments, he would walk up to old ladies and say, "You look so nice today." And he had no inhibitions about going up to a stranger who was sick and start praying for them. At home, if Susan wasn't feeling well, he would go outside and suddenly come back with a handful of dandelions with the dirt still hanging off it to give to her. 'Feel better, mommy,' he would tell her. If he was in a store, and if someone standing in front of us didn't have enough change, he would whip some out of his pocket and give it to them. He couldn't even count yet—he simply gave them whatever he had jingling in his pocket. He just made everyone smile. He never got angry or bitter over his condition. Justin should have been a priest. He was the kind of person who just had a heart for everybody and cared so much about people.

As for our daughter Kirstin, while she felt sorry for everything that was happening to her brothers, she also felt left out and even jealous over all the time they were receiving from Susan and me. We would find out later that she was angry at us over that lack of attention. It's so hard being young parents and having a couple of sick ones and another child who's healthy. The natural thinking is that you don't have to pay the healthy child as much attention.

But we were wrong there. And if we had to do it all over again, we would have tried to do better by her.

It was a constant struggle on so many fronts. We had issues in the family unit, and we still have issues. Being a Christian doesn't make you perfect. I still mess up. I start every day with, "Lord, forgive me." And every night, and two or three times during the day, I'll pray to God, "Forgive me and cleanse me from inside out." Because I don't know if I offended somebody by the way I looked at them or from the way I said something. And I thank God that He judges me and not people—and that He knows my heart.

On August 30, 1982, Timothy endured a 12-hour surgery on his eye at Massachusetts Eye and Ear that began very early that morning. He came out of surgery at around 4:00 PM that afternoon. I had a 7:35 PM game at Fenway that night against the A's, so I needed to go. As I got ready to leave his hospital room, I kissed him on the forehead and said, "Tim, I love you. I've got to go to the ballpark now. I'm late. Batting practice starts in an hour." Still quite groggy and barely able to talk after the surgery, Timothy said softly, "Dad, I love you, too. Can you do me a favor?" I said, "Sure, Tim what's that?" And he asked, "Can you hit me a home run tonight?" Realizing how difficult a promise that would be to keep, but needing to leave, I said, "Okay, Tim, I'll try." As I got to the door, he said, "Dad, Dad, can you do me another favor?" I said, "What's that, Tim?" And he asked, "Can you hit me *two* home runs tonight?" Again, needing to go, I exhaled and said, "Okay, okay, Tim, I'll try. I'll try." And as God is my judge, after that emotionally exhausting day, I hit *two home runs*—and a triple for good measure—in one of the best games of my life! That's how God works—it was unbelievable! After I hit the second one and was rounding the bases, I looked up to the sky and went, "Thank you." Timothy was watching the game on television with Susan in his hospital room and could see the lights of Fenway Park from his window, making it even more special. When I got back to the hospital, he was very tired but just so happy I had hit two home runs for him. I think I was even happier than he was. If there was ever a spiritual moment in my life, that was it. I only wish he had asked me to hit 400 more!

Another time that same season, the Red Sox PR guy, Dick Bresciani, asked me to say hello to a very sick boy named Dan who had liver cancer. Dick told me he had stopped chemotherapy and had lost the will to live. So I brought him into the clubhouse, signed a bat and some baseballs for him, and took him around to introduce him to some of the guys. At the end of his visit, I took him back out to his parents, and he said, "Dewey, would you do me a favor?" I said, "What's that, Dan?" Acting a little shy, he said, "Would you hit me a home run tonight?" Again, knowing what a difficult promise that would be to keep, I said, "Well, Dan, if I hit one tonight, it will be for you." And I did it again!

But the story gets better. After my encounter with Dan, I never knew what happened to him. Fast-forward 20 years and Dick calls me and says, "Do you remember Dan—the boy who had liver cancer? Well, he's still alive! NESN is shooting a story about it and would like you to come up to Boston to be a part of it." So, on the day of shooting at Fenway, Dan, now in his late thirties, was standing with his brother by the Red Sox dugout, looked directly into one of the NESN cameras, and said, "Hey, Dewey, hit one over the net!" He didn't know I was coming, so when I suddenly appeared, he did a double-take and started crying like a baby. He gave me a huge hug in what was such a special, emotional moment. The home run I hit for Dan inspired him to live and go through treatment—and he beat cancer!

Those were the "promised" home runs I can document. But I know there were other instances later in my career when it happened, because a few of the many young people I visited in hospitals came up to me later and would say things like, "Thank you. That home run you hit meant so much to me." Those home runs gave me a sense of how much a ballplayer can influence, encourage, and help people in need. I only wish I had done more—especially for those who needed inspiration the most.

CHAPTER 14

A NEW DAWN

THERE WERE NUMEROUS REASONS for optimism as the 1984 season got underway. After years of losing star players via free agency, and after a failed coup attempt by a group led by Buddy LeRoux to wrestle majority ownership of the Red Sox away from Jean Yawkey, the club was again spending like a big-market team in the tradition of Tom Yawkey. As a result, guys like Rice, Bob Stanley, and myself—part of the veteran nucleus going forward—were soon taken care of with lucrative, long-term deals. The dark clouds that had hovered over the organization for years had finally cleared.

I could also begin to see the base of our club's future come together. The pitching staff would soon be anchored by Roger Clemens, our first-round pick in the amateur draft the year before. He would be promoted to the big-league roster that season and show glimpses of the greatness that was to come from his special right arm. Little did we know at the time just how incredible Clemens would turn out to be. Oil Can Boyd and Bruce Hurst were the young workhorses of the pitching staff. And the versatile Al Nipper was one of those guys you could bring in from the bullpen and he'd put out a fire, or you could spot-start him. Either way, he'd pitch his rear-end off for you. That pitching core gave us confidence that our team could compete against anybody.

Offensively, we had the most lethal outfield in baseball that season, with Rice, Tony Armas, and me all driving in more than 100 runs. Rich Gedman had developed into one of the best-hitting catchers in all of baseball, and Mike Easler had a big year as our designated hitter. Marty Barrett, in his first full season as our regular second baseman, hit .303. And in just his third major league season, Wade Boggs had established himself as one of the elite hitters in the game. There wasn't a weak spot in the lineup.

It was hard to comprehend the level of success Boggs had at the plate from the time he came up in 1982. In his rookie year, he batted .349; in his second year, he hit a league-leading .361; and then he batted .325 in his '84 campaign before going on a streak of winning the batting crown in the next four straight seasons. His numbers were better at the big-league level than what he produced during his six years in the minor leagues. And his on-base percentage was off the charts before that was considered an important statistic. Boggs' ability to square the ball up was incredible. He was just so disciplined—not only with pitch location, but also where he hit the ball on the field. I rarely saw him pull the ball in games, yet in batting practice, he could hit home run after home run to right field and center field all day long. During games, he stayed within his routine of hitting the ball primarily from center to left field—his strength—and that's what made him so successful. And it's also what made it so ironic that his 3,000[th] hit was a home run deep into the right field stands in Tampa Bay. He could hit the ball wherever he wanted with authority. He was that great and was special to watch.

Wade also worked hard at his defense as a third baseman. He was not a great defender when he came up but turned himself into one, winning two Gold Glove Awards later in his career as a Yankee to become a complete ballplayer.

We would pick up yet another big bat in a late-May trade with the Chicago Cubs for Bill Buckner. We dealt my dear friend Dennis Eckersley in the trade, which involved two elite players who perhaps needed a change of venue. Eck had struggled with an ERA north of five over the last season and a half, and Buck started the first third of the '84 season hitting just .209 in limited action for the Cubs.

Ironically, much like how I hit it off with Eck immediately after we traded for him in '78, Buck and I also connected right away. The admiration was immediate, and it was special. I absolutely loved him. He was a gamer and made the game fun for me again. One of the things I loved most about Buck was his personality. It was just so contagious. What made his pleasant demeanor even more impressive was knowing how much pain and discomfort he was always in. One of his ankles was pretty much fused together and was bigger than the other one. But if Buck hit a soft grounder to the infield and smelled a hit, suddenly he could turn on the burners with the best of them. He still had great speed when he needed it. That was the gamer in him. But as soon as he hit the first base bag, he'd go into that limp he had. And then he'd steal second! He was fun. Before he tore up his ankle, he was a base-stealing threat with the Dodgers, stealing 28 bases for them in '76.

In a brotherly way, Buck also knew when to put me in my place. One evening after a day game in Detroit, we went out and had a nice dinner together. As we were walking back to the Pontchartrain Hotel, where the team was staying, we ran into one of the Tigers pitchers and his wife. I took one look at the woman and noticed a glow about her. She looked to me like she could be carrying a child. Usually, I'm like 99 percent right on this stuff. So, after a few minutes, I asked her innocently, "How far along are you?" But she responded, "I'm *not* pregnant." So that kind of cut short the conversation right there. They went on their way, and we went on ours. Buck did nothing the rest of the way back to the Pontchartrain but just pound my left arm with his left fist. Just *pounding* it. "You idiot!" he said. "They're *separated*! She flew in to see him to try to get their marriage back together. And you said *that*?" It was something that Kramer might have said on *Seinfeld*. I couldn't say anything, so I just let Buck beat me up on the street. I deserved every minute of it.

One of the things we did was eat together on the road—often with Barrett. The three of us went on this diet that Buck had introduced us to, called "Eat to Win!" It was basically a diet high in pasta and carbohydrates and low in fat. The thing that stood out most about the diet was how we couldn't eat sugar. I couldn't believe all the foods that contained sugar. Even ketchup uses it as an ingredient. Well, I went on a 1-for-21 slump during the diet and, during a homestand, I was so upset about it that I was lying in bed at 1:00 AM, unable to fall asleep. I kept trying to figure out my swing and how to break out of the slump. Feeling restless, I got out of bed, went downstairs to the kitchen, opened the freezer door, and took out a pint of Häagen-Dazs Rum Raisin ice cream. At first, I took just a spoonful, but then I ended up devouring the whole pint. Because I hadn't eaten sugar in three months, my eyes were wide-open at five in the morning thanks to a sugar high I can't even describe. I finally drifted off around 9:00 AM and slept for about four hours. Luckily, the slump didn't last too much longer.

As for Barrett, even though he was still a young player at that time, he fit right in with Buck and me. He was intelligent beyond his years in so many ways. Marty was a blue-collar type of player, working hard at everything—baserunning, arm-strength, fielding, hitting—to get the most out of his abilities. And he would give me hand signals of the signs behind his back when playing second base so I could get a feel if the hitter might be out in front of the ball or a little late—that type of thing. Buck and I respected his work ethic and baseball intellect.

When Marty wasn't having dinner with us on the road, he would often play cards with some of the other guys to wind down after games—and he usually won. He was so mentally quick and bright that I wouldn't doubt if he was a card counter. He'd probably be banned in Las Vegas or Atlantic City because he was such a great card player.

I was more than happy to mentor him on things unrelated to baseball. When we would go golfing, grab a meal, or sit together on the team bus, he picked my brain about business and finances, always running ideas by me. In the mid-'80s, he knew I was flipping homes before it became popular with the help of a dear friend in Boston. I preached to Marty my philosophy of the "Four F's" of real estate investing: *Find it, Finance it, Fix it, and Flip it.* He really took to that and ever since he retired, he's been buying homes, renting them, selling them, flipping them. Every time I talk to Marty, he's in a different house. Most importantly, he learned how to buy homes in desirable areas. At one time, he owned 30 rental properties in Las Vegas. He really listened to what I was telling him and has done extremely well in real estate. Marty was always smarter than the average bear. He is one of those guys that was smart in school but was also street smart—a rare quality. Sometimes you find somebody who's so intelligent, they don't know left from right and don't know how to survive. Marty knew not only how to survive but thrive. I am glad to know my advice to him had a big impact on his financial life.

Another way I mentored Barrett was in how to deal with the press. His locker was next to mine and the main thing I impressed upon him was when you're talking to a reporter about another player, pretend that player is sitting right next to you. So, if you wouldn't say something to that player's face, you wouldn't say it to a media member. You'd always stick up for your teammates unless your teammates disrespected you—which almost never happens. I learned that from Yaz years before. I also tried to give my teammates credit whenever I could with reporters. If I hit a three-run homer, I would say something like, "Well, if Marty didn't get a walk and Buckner didn't get on base, I wouldn't have hit that three-run homer." And Barrett was like a sponge, adopting much of what he observed from me and putting it into everyday practice. I always tried to be like a big brother to him and he's remained a dear friend to this day.

In fact, I tried to become more of a leader to all the younger guys on the club, especially after Yaz's retirement the year before. Even Susan got into the act, going out of her way to help their wives adjust to big-league life through self-preservation. Realizing what a tough environment it could be on them, her standard advice was, "Don't share too much personal information with others. Just keep things simple and you'll be just fine." She especially helped Holly Hurst, a sweet and wonderful woman, and a few of the other wives know where the "landmines" were. It's not easy being a baseball wife. You have to work hard to fulfill almost all of the family responsibilities largely on your own while not resenting your husband's life in the spotlight. You have to accept it all to make everything work. And Susan did that, while doing a great job of keeping me in the kids' lives while I travelled during the season. Aside from turning the games on television and telling them, "There's Daddy on TV," she kept growth calendars of me holding a glass of milk and a baseball bat in their rooms. She would sometimes forget they were there, and they would scare the life out of her every time! But she kept me in the picture, which was so important to all of us.

Susan and the kids were no strangers to the ballpark, making the trip to Fenway whenever their schedules permitted. One of those visits was especially memorable. After the Celtics won the '84 NBA Finals over the Los Angeles Lakers that June, the kids enjoyed a real treat when Celtics center Robert "the Chief" Parish, as great a basketball player as he was a gentleman, visited our clubhouse. Standing very quietly in a suit and tie against one of the pillars, at 7'1", his presence and stature were awe-inspiring. Justin was by my locker and twiddling his thumbs. I could tell he was kind of in a thinking mode. As I was getting changed into my uniform, the next thing I know, Justin, just six years old at the time, was now standing directly in front of Robert. Still twiddling his thumbs, he looked down at his feet before looking up at him and innocently asked—as only a small child missing his two front teeth with a lisp could—"What *twibe* are you from?" Robert, being the classy individual he was, just started laughing. I was appalled because I didn't think he'd come out with something like that, but little did I know that he had been studying different tribes in Africa in school. So asking Robert what tribe he was from just naively came out of his mouth. Justin always was so honest with his thoughts. And the Chief was and still is a good man for his understanding. I'll never forget that as long as I live.

————————

From a personal standpoint, I had a great '84 campaign. I led the American League in OPS and runs scored and belted 32 home runs with 104 RBIs while winning my seventh Gold Glove Award. I also hit the only cycle of my career on June 28, capping off the day with a three-run walk-off home run in the 11th inning.

Another thing I started doing more of was swinging away on 3-and-0 counts—with the help of a little acting. I would look down at the third base coach and shrug my shoulders disappointingly, and go, *Really?* to make the opposition think, by my body language, that the take-sign was on. I ended up with a bunch of 3-and-0 home runs that season, never getting cheated. Anybody that swings 3-and-0 and hits one off the end of the bat or pops it up shouldn't swing 3-and-0. If you're going to swing in that situation, you better make solid contact. You've got to stay within yourself and only look for a pitch in a certain area. And if it was there, I would put my "A" swing on it. The older I got, the better I got at hitting 3-and-0.

With all the success I was having at the plate that season, the bleacher crowd took notice. Many times, after hitting a big home run, as I trotted back out to my position in right field the following inning, the fans out there would rise in unison and cheer me on. I would always acknowledge the crowd for doing that, tipping my cap right back to them. The feeling I would get from that remains one of my fondest memories of playing at Fenway. It exemplified how great the fans are in New England and how much they respect players who really bust their rear end. Terry O'Reilly of the Bruins was a great example of the Boston fans' adulation for hard-nosed play. O'Reilly was not a great skater, but nobody on the ice worked harder, fought more, and had a bigger heart than he did. And the fans knew that. They "got" what O'Reilly was all about and showed him their appreciation with rousing ovations.

But what was most important to me about the '84 season was the leap the team took over the previous season. We finished with 86 wins, an eight-game improvement. But no matter how well we played, no team in the AL East—the toughest division in baseball at that time—was going to catch a historically great Detroit Tigers club that held a firm grasp on first place the entire season on their way to a World Series championship. Still, we felt encouraged by the team we had put together and believed the '85 campaign could be a special one.

We opened the '85 campaign with a three-game series against the Yankees at Fenway Park a day after a foot of snow had fallen in Boston. But on that morning, the sun was shining brightly, the snow had all but melted, and like most games against the Yankees, there was a buzz in the ballpark. Every time we played the Yankees was big and it was always overhyped by the media. There would be more cameras, reporters, and talk show types than any other games just because the Yankees were in town. And the fans were really into it. As a player, I wanted to beat every team equally, but our fans only cared about beating the Yankees. It's all many of them cared about. And what made the contests even more fierce in '85 was how stacked both of our lineups were. The top of the Yankees lineup was tremendous with Rickey Henderson, Willie Randolph, Don Mattingly, Dave Winfield, and Don Baylor. But ours was just as impressive, which made for a great matchup. So, the tremendous hype generated not only because it was opening day, but also a game against the Yankees, was felt all over town. The rivalry, particularly for the fans, may have been the biggest in all of sports.

What on paper should have been a balanced series was a one-sided rout as we hammered the Yankees' pitching for 29 runs over those three games behind strong pitching performances from Boyd, Hurst, and Clemens. Sweeping the Yankees and then winning our fourth game of the season over the White Sox seemed like a good omen. But that enthusiasm dimmed when significant injuries to Clemens, Rice, Armas, and Nipper really extinguished any chance we had of catching the Toronto Blue Jays and their 99 wins.

Personally, I led the team in home runs, but I was just as pleased with my .378 on-base percentage, which included a league-leading 114 walks. It showed me that my discipline at the plate was where it needed to be. I also won my eighth Gold Glove

Award in 10 seasons, so a trophy shelf the length of a wall in my house was really filling up. But again, team results *always* meant more to me than my individual accomplishments. And despite the .500 record we had in '85, I knew that as our club continued to mature, and if we stayed healthy, we could be as good as any club in baseball. And I was really encouraged by how well we played late in the season—going 19–9 in September—despite being out of the race and having nothing to play for at that point. I thought that showed the character and talent that we had and it boded well for the '86 season.

CHAPTER 15

RETURN TO GLORY

IN THE VERY BEST OF WAYS, there was a different look and feel to the club as we broke spring training camp in '86. Clemens, still an unheralded pitcher with unlimited potential, was back in the rotation after getting shut down during the previous season due to a small flap tear that kept getting caught in his rotator cuff joint. Any surgery performed on a pitcher's arm—their *livelihood*—has the potential for disaster, but credit Dr. James Andrews with fixing Rocket up and setting the stage for a pitching performance for the ages.

Another highly significant development occurred late that spring training when we acquired Don Baylor in a trade with the Yankees in exchange for Mike Easler. That was a total game-changer in terms of our mindset—the final, missing piece of the puzzle for us. We already had so many stars, but when we got Baylor, I thought to myself, *We can win this thing.* Not only was Baylor a former AL MVP and one of the premier sluggers in the game who we could stick in the heart of our lineup, but he was also a true leader on the field and in the clubhouse.

Having Baylor changed the whole demeanor of our ball club just by his presence. Right away, he assumed the role of judge of a "kangaroo court" he established with the team. At our so-called "proceedings," he put on a gray wig like Thomas Jefferson, had a gavel to signal for order in the court, and just fired verdicts and fines down on everybody for committing baseball crimes like mental mistakes, being late for batting practice, fraternizing with the opposition—things like that. The fines were small and more symbolic, ranging from $20 to $50, but if you dared challenge "the Judge," he would slam the gavel down and double your fine. But he had a way of doing it that was fun and brought a greater unity to the ball club. "Judge Baylor" would collect thousands of dollars that season and put it to good use. On an off night during a West Coast trip, he rented a magnificent Seattle home with an incredible view of the Space Needle for a team party, which was truly unforgettable. Baylor would quickly become one of the greatest teammates—and friends—I ever had in baseball.

With a couple of weeks left in spring training, our manager, John McNamara, called me into his office. "Our leadoff hitter doesn't want to lead off," he said. "Would you like to lead off?" "Whatever you want me to do," I replied. A couple of nights later, I had a dream that I was going to start off our season with a home run. It was such a vivid premonition that I started telling people close to me about it—first Susan, then Marty Barrett, and then—probably a mistake—our hitting coach, Walt Hriniak. Upon telling Walt, he turned and walked away, then came right back and kind of pushed me in the chest with his arms like Elaine would do to people on Seinfeld. "I *don't* want you thinking home run," he said sternly.

Hriniak was a firm believer that if you thought home run, you would get too big with your swing and your head wouldn't stay down. If you just thought base hit, then the home runs would come on their own. Even after I hit a home run, he would come up to me and say something like, "What are you going to do next time up?" And I would always reply with, "I'm going to hit a line drive." "Dynamite!" he'd exclaim. He always wanted to make sure I didn't get out of control with my swing and that my head didn't fly out. The more your head stayed down, the better chance you had of hitting the ball hard and getting a hit. That's why even after I hit two home runs in a game, I never tried to hit a third one. If I had, it would have totally messed me up.

I loved Walt and how dedicated he was with his students. When you were working in the cage with him, there was no one more important than you. People would come by and try to talk with him, and he was like, "Not now! Go watch some film. Come back later!"

Opening Day in Detroit—the moment of truth had finally arrived. Before a sell-out crowd, I was getting anxious—*really* anxious. There was never a time in my 10,569 career plate appearances when I didn't have butterflies, but leading off on Opening Day against future Hall of Fame pitcher Jack Morris had me jumping up and down to try to remain calm. After the national anthem ended, I looked up into the stands, and the crowd was going nuts—totally pumped up. As I walked toward the bat rack in the dugout, Walt said to me, "What are you going to do up there?" And I said, "Walt, I'm going to hit a line drive to right center." "Dynamite, that's what I want to hear!" he said.

But as I started walking up the dugout steps to the on-deck circle, I turned to Barrett and said, "I'm going deep on the first pitch!" Morris had a great forkball and an excellent slider, but I was looking for a belt-high fastball right down the middle on the first pitch because I knew, even though Jack was a veteran, he probably had Opening Day jitters, too, and I wanted to get ahead in the count.

After Morris finished his warm-up pitches, I slammed my bat to the ground so the donut could come flying off and made my way to the batter's box. I just kept repeating in my head, "He's coming in there with a fastball." I got into my batting stance and looked out at Morris, and he wound up and threw an elevated fastball—a little out of my zone—but I unloaded on it, sending the pitch high and deep over the 400-foot sign in centerfield for a home run—just like in the dream! It happened! It happened! When I hit it, no one was more taken aback than me. Morris had a look on his face like, *Are you kidding me?* As I touched first base, I was just like, *Thank you, Lord! Thank you! This is unbelievable. None of the guys, except Marty, is ever going to believe this story. No one!* I was just floating around the bases. It was such a special moment in my career and a great way to start the season.

A few weeks later, on April 29, an especially cold and damp night at Fenway, we played the seminal game of the young season that would set the tone for the rest of the campaign. It was on that night that Clemens stunned the baseball world by setting the major league record with 20 strikeouts in a nine-inning game over the Seattle Mariners. He was so dominant that the Mariners were barely even fouling balls off, as there were mostly swings-and-misses and called strikes against them. To achieve what he did less than a month into the season after coming back from surgery was remarkable.

Interestingly enough, Rocket was actually *losing* that game 1–0 after giving up a solo home run to Gorman Thomas with two outs in the top of the seventh inning. The opposing pitcher, Mike Moore, was pitching a gem himself. But I was able to contribute to Roger's big night with a three-run homer deep into the centerfield bleachers—against the wind—off Moore in the bottom of the inning to give Roger all the margin he would need in our 3–1 victory.

After the game, we were all talking about how Baylor dropped a pop-up in foul territory in the fourth inning, giving Clemens a chance to strike him out—which he did. But it was all in fun.

The reality was we were all celebrating this *special* moment, this *Red Sox* moment, and this *baseball* moment in history. The 20 strikeouts were simply monumental. We all just held our heads a little bit higher as a team after that game. It was a real character builder for us. As for Roger, I can only imagine what it did for his confidence, especially after coming back from the surgery. Clemens was now 4–0, clearly our ace, with Hurst, Boyd, and Nipper filling out the rest of a formidable rotation. We felt the possibilities were limitless for us now.

By late June, we held an eight-game lead in the AL East with the trade deadline approaching. What often happens at the deadline is the good teams look to improve themselves while the struggling clubs look to unload some of their stars to build for the future. So when our front office saw the opportunity to trade for an all-time great pitcher, it did just that. On June 29, we acquired Tom Seaver from the struggling Chicago White Sox in exchange for our young backup centerfielder, Steve Lyons.

Seaver may have been 41 and, as it would turn out, in his last major league season, but he could still pitch and had a tremendous baseball mind that would serve our young pitching staff well. We lockered next to one another and had many conversations about pitching. He talked to me about how he would throw pitches in certain areas of the plate just to watch the hitter's reaction. For example, if he was facing a right-handed hitter, he might throw a slider low and away for a ball because he wanted to see how that hitter responded to it. If the batter went for it with his left shoulder closed and staying on the pitch, then Seaver's mindset was, *I know I can now get him out up and in.* And if the right-handed hitter's left shoulder kind of opened up a little bit, then Seaver knew he could get him out down and away. That was the kind of higher-level knowledge Seaver would pass on to Clemens and Hurst. I don't know anything about pitching other than what

I didn't like to see as a hitter when I played. That's really as far as my pitching knowledge goes. But for Seaver to explain this to me was pretty impressive. He was a great student of the game.

Like most any pennant-contending team, we would be the beneficiary of some of the craziest finishes to games I ever witnessed. The first one occurred on May 19 with the Minnesota Twins leading us 7–6 with two outs and nobody on base in the bottom of the ninth at Fenway. Twins' pitcher Ron Davis walked Barrett, and then Boggs followed with a double, and Buckner was intentionally walked to load the bases. Rice walked to bring in Barrett with the tying run, and then Marc Sullivan gets hit in the butt to win the game 8–7!

Then on May 27, in something right out of the *Twilight Zone*, the famous "Fog Game" came to pass. We were playing at Cleveland's old Municipal Stadium, the so-called "Mistake by the Lake," when a heavy, thick fog rolled in off Lake Erie. We were leading 2–0 in the bottom of the sixth, but the Indians were threatening with two men on and two outs. It was at that point that crew chief Larry Barnett called for a fog delay. The umpires called us off the field for about 15 minutes, but the fog was still there. To test visibility to see if the game could be continued, the umpires asked Bobby Bonds, then the batting coach for the Indians, to hit me some fungoes. The umpires figured having representatives from both teams involved with this test was fair and equitable. Well, knowing we had a 2–0 lead and that the game would be called if we couldn't go on, I had a little Hollywood in me that day. Hurst described me as looking like a dancing bear trying to catch the fly balls before letting them land 5 or 10 feet from me. I'd cover my head like they were going to hit me on the noggin.

But I could see the balls fine—I just acted like I couldn't. And that's when one of the umpires came out to the outfield, put up a big safe sign, and said, "Game's over! That's it!" They called the game right there. I jogged back into the dugout and told my teammates, "Boys, we're going home."

Back in the clubhouse, on the other side of my locker, was Oil Can. I can remember a reporter asking him, "Have you ever seen anything like this before, Oil Can?" And he goes, "I've never seen anything like it. But that's what you get for building a ballpark by the *ocean*." I was getting undressed and getting ready for the shower when I heard this and went, "What'd you say, Can?" And I just walked away laughing, shaking my head. You can't make that up. Just a classic thing for him to say. It was like a Yogi-ism.

By the time we left the ballpark to get on the team bus, maybe 40 minutes later, there was not a cloud in the sky. The stars were glowing. It was as clear as could be. The fog had rolled completely out of the area. But by that point, of course, they couldn't bring us back into the ballpark to continue the game. It was over.

Another bizarre ending happened on June 10 during a 3–3 tie game against the Toronto Blue Jays. We had two outs with the bases loaded in the top of the ninth when Barrett walked halfway to the batter's box, then turned back around to the dugout and told McNamara he didn't hit Blue Jays' reliever Mark Eichhorn very well, advising him to utilize little-used Mike Stenhouse to bat for him in that very big spot. It was a highly unconventional move. Stenhouse would work the count full before drawing a walk to force in the go-ahead run in a game we would hold on to win 4–3. It was Stenhouse's only RBI of the season and the last of his short big-league career.

A month later, on July 10, perhaps our most outlandish comeback occurred in the bottom of the 12th at Fenway in a game against the California Angels. With the Angels leading 7–4 and with us down to our last out, Rice cracked a two-run homer to cut the lead to 7–6. But it looked like our night was done when Baylor popped a ball up to third base and the sure-handed Rick Burleson dropped the ball—which blew my mind—to allow Don to reach first. After I walked, we had runners on first and second. Rich Gedman then singled to right field to score Baylor to tie the game at 7–7 as Geddy and I advanced to second and third on a throwing error by Angels first baseman Wally Joyner. The Angels then brought in Todd Fischer to relieve Mike Cook, and Fischer *balked* me home with the winning run! I can still see Angels catcher Bob Boone jumping up and down, arguing with home plate umpire Joe Brinkman over the call.

These were the types of quirky victories you need over the course of a long season to win a pennant. Unless you're just some All-Star team that is a powerhouse, you have to get some breaks. And fortunately for us, we certainly had our share of memorable ones.

By the All-Star break in mid-July, we held a seven-game lead in the AL East. It was already shaping up to be a special kind of year and was incredible in so many ways. When you're playing well, everyone plays together, everyone works together, and everyone's on the same page. As a result, everyone's happier. Any kind of situation that would normally ruffle your feathers no longer does. Even your travel is better. Your charter flight gets delayed, you arrive in town at 4:00 AM, and there's no bus. No problem! You're like, *Hey, it's okay. The bus will get here eventually.* Winning just makes everything better.

A by-product of winning is the clubhouse hijinks that take place. And part of the fun for me was giving hot foots. I admit that I took great pride in the practice. I learned from the prank-sters of old—watching Yaz and pitcher Gary Peters perform the act shortly after I came up to the big leagues. It was harmless stuff—nobody ever got hurt.

One of my best hot foots took place in Detroit in early August. The recipient was the beloved Johnny Pesky, at that time a special instructor who often suited up before games to work with our players. Pesky may have been 67 years old then, but he was still a fiery, aggressive individual. Anyway, before one of the Tigers games, Johnny was playing cards in the clubhouse with some of the guys—sitting on a stool with a towel on top of it. Johnny was in his underwear, with his top, socks, and cleats on. He would pull the elastic from his socks over his cleats and always put his pants on last. It must have been a thing they did in the 1940s when he played. So, I had the bright idea of giving him a hot foot. His feet were under his stool, he's got his elbows on his knees, he's looking down at his cards, and he's not paying any attention to his surroundings. I lit a cigarette and then wrapped six match heads with bubble gum around it. Once the cigarette got close enough to the match heads, it would explode into a flame.

I quietly got on my knees and went under his stool from behind him, and affixed the cigarette on to his right sole by his little toe where your foot really presses against it. I'm watching as it's get-ting warmer and warmer while Johnny continues to play cards. Other guys were walking by, seeing what was going on, and tried to distract Pesky—looking at his and the other players' cards—so he wouldn't notice what I had done. It was classic—something you wish you could have recorded. Then, after about 10 minutes, it went off and there was a good six inches of flame coming from his foot. I saw it and started laughing because Johnny was such a red ass. He grabbed his stool and threw it up against the lockers—not caring in the least if it hit anybody. He took the towel that had been under the stool and put out the fire. Pesky was so pissed. He had fire in his eyes and wanted to kill somebody. But it was all in fun, everybody started laughing, and Johnny eventually let it go.

However, later that month, I inadvertently went too far. We returned to Boston from a road trip with our division lead reduced to just four games. Rene Lachemann, our third base coach, was sitting by his locker with his head in his hands, elbows on his knees, and rubbing his hands in a woe-is-me kind of way. He just looked so depressed. We had to do something to get him going. What we didn't know at the time was how "Lach" had just put a new roof on his home in Phoenix, thinking we were a lock for the playoffs. All the extra postseason money he was counting on was suddenly disappearing.

So, I came up with one of my "brilliant" ideas. I pushed a spittoon underneath his chair without him noticing it, put some rubbing alcohol on a big ball of paper the size of a soccer ball, tossed it inside, and lit a match to ignite it. To my amazement, the flames went three feet above each side of his chair—singeing some of his hair. I was like, *Oh my gosh, what did I do?!* Lach, a great guy, was mad as could be. He grabbed the chair and fired it up above the lockers off the wall. He was swearing and shouting, "Who did that?! Who's man enough to do that?! Let's go! Let's go!"

I had to step forward and said, "Lach, I did it." So, he pushed me, and I pushed back, warning him, "Don't push me, Lach." But he proceeded to throw a haymaker over the top right of me. Well, I was into Martial Arts karate for about six years back then, so I blocked it, grabbed his right arm, and threw him on the ground. I started pounding on his head—just beating the pulp out of him. Bruce Hurst, such a sensitive soul, was there holding a banana, kind of sobbing, and said, "Dewey, stop hitting Lach!" One of our relievers, Steve Crawford, a mountain of a man from Oklahoma who stood 6'5" and 240 pounds, rushed over and, with just his left hand, picked me up off the floor by my belt. I'm flailing like a little kid—my legs and arms are flopping everywhere. Crawford, in his Oklahoma regionalism goes, "Dewey, you stop hitting Lach." And then he goes to Lach, "Now you just stay down there." Of course, Lach wasn't going anywhere. So, that ended the skirmish. I really felt awful about everything and apologized to Lach afterward. But I had this thing that went back to my days fighting as a boy in school—never take a swing at me. Push me and I'm coming right back at you. Lach and I made up and we've remained good friends ever since. When you're together with 25 guys for eight and a half months, you're like brothers and you're liable to disagree and fight with one another from time to time. That's how it was. Thankfully, we started winning again, and Lach was feeling better about buying his new roof.

One of the reasons we got back to our winning ways was due to a trade we made with the Seattle Mariners on August 17 when we acquired shortstop Spike Owen and center fielder Dave Henderson in exchange for Rey Quiñones and three players to be named later. It was nothing short of a *steal* for us.

In Spike, we received a solid shortstop—quick hands, great glove, and good speed. He was a real sparkplug and fit in with us right away. It was a little hard to understand why the Mariners would deal their team captain who was still a relatively young player at just 25 years old. My only theory was that Spike was coming up on free agency and the Mariners wanted to get whatever they could for him.

With "Hendu," we acquired a *tremendous* athlete—a freak of nature. Dave was a chiseled 220 pounds yet never lifted a weight. His athleticism was such that he could jump sideways from the dugout floor up to the top step. He was a great centerfielder and was one of my all-time favorite teammates. He always had a smile on his face with that huge, gap-toothed grin of his that was simply contagious. He had more fun playing the game than anybody I ever saw.

And to tell you what kind of a devoted man he was, when he and his wife divorced, he took custody and cared for their two boys—including his eldest son, Chase, who suffered from Angelman Syndrome, a rare genetic disorder that impacts the nervous system. I was deeply saddened when Hendu died of a heart attack in 2015 at just 57 years old. I miss him very much.

When we got Hendu, I didn't know where he would fit in. Tony Armas was our centerfielder—and a good one. But he was bothered by leg injuries at various times during the season and the Red Sox felt Hendu would be a good insurance policy if Tony couldn't play all the time. That thinking by management would prove to be prophetic and pay dividends for us almost immediately.

An 11-game winning streak that began in late August and ran well into September helped us pull away from the pack and increase our division lead to a season-high 10½ games. It was now just a matter of time before we would clinch our first title since 1975. And on a sunny Sunday afternoon on September 28th at Fenway, we would finish the job. Oil Can would go the distance in our 12–3 victory over the Blue Jays. The last out was caught, appropriately enough, by Buckner near first base. He tried to jump up and down like the rest of us but didn't have much spring left in his step. Still, he was like a seven-year-old kid, just as happy as could be.

During that final half inning of the division clincher, so many emotions were running through my head. I thought back to how after '75, when I was just 23 years old, I was so sure we would win four or five more pennants and have a good shot at winning a couple of world championships. It was baffling to me how that didn't happen with some of the strong teams and great players we had—particularly in '77 and '78. But then I thought about how

Hall of Famers like Ernie Banks and Billy Williams never played in a World Series and how hard it is to get there. And there were many other all-time greats that never even made it to the playoffs, much less the Fall Classic. It gave me perspective of how difficult this game can be and how you have to appreciate the glorious moments like this one when you can.

After 11 years, we were finally going back to the postseason with another shot at a world championship. The long wait made it extra sweet in many ways. It's hard to explain the fulfillment and all the hard work that went into that joyous moment in time. It was an unbelievable feeling—a dream come true I yearned for more than a decade to happen.

CHAPTER 16

ONE FOR THE AGES

T HE ANGELS AND THEIR 64,223 FANS were ready to go crazy. Ahead three games to one in the ALCS and leading 5–2 in Game 5 as we batted in the top of the ninth, they were just three outs away from making their first trip to the World Series in franchise history. The stadium became fully enclosed six years earlier for Rams football, adding an additional 23,000 seats and making it one of the largest and loudest stadiums in the country when at full capacity. And that ninth inning was no exception. The decibel level was so high, it hurt my ears to the point where I had to put earplugs in.

Through eight innings, Angels' pitcher Mike Witt was outstanding, allowing just two runs on six hits. And he was still going strong as he started the ninth. After giving up a leadoff single to Buckner that barely made it through the infield, he struck out Rice looking on three pitches. The Angels were now just two outs away. Much of the sell-out crowd began moving down toward field level, preparing to pour on to the field after the final out. The stadium police began positioning themselves in our dugout and around the outer edges of foul territory to control the crowd.

Witt would get ahead of our next hitter, Baylor, 1-2, before Don laid off of two really tough pitches to run the count full. Either pitch would have prompted most hitters to chase them, but Baylor had such great discipline at the plate he was able to lay off both of them. Don would reach out for the next pitch—down and away—and with his exceptional strength hit one just beyond the reach of centerfielder Gary Pettis and over the fence to cut the Angels' lead to 5–4.

That brought me to the plate now representing the tying run. I kept reminding myself to not be overanxious and to get a good pitch to drive somewhere. Witt's first two pitches were on the outside corner for strikes, though I thought the second one—a fastball—was at least an inch or so off the plate and I let home plate umpire Rocky Roe know it. Now down 0-2 in the count, I had to protect the plate and swing at anything close. The next pitch was a slow breaking ball that Witt got up, but I just missed hitting is squarely, popping out to Doug DeCinces at third base. We were now down to our final out. Our magnificent season and everything we worked so hard for over the last six months now hung in the balance.

But we still had hope because Gedman had crushed the ball in all three of his at-bats against Witt—first a two-run homer to right field, then a double to deep left-center, and finally a line drive single to right field. With that in mind, Angels' manager Gene Mauch made the highly debatable move of relieving Witt, who had otherwise been so masterful against the rest of our lineup, with left-handed reliever Gary Lucas. Mauch had apparently seen enough of Gedman bashing balls all over the park off Witt and saw Lucas—in a left-handed pitcher versus left-handed hitter scenario—as a better alternative.

Mauch was a great manager and an excellent strategist. In his defense, I don't know how anybody could have second-guessed his decision to bring in Lucas. But what Mauch couldn't control was the execution of his players. So when Lucas plunked Geddy with a high fastball on his first pitch, it changed everything. Now we had the tying run on base and potential winning run at the plate in Dave Henderson.

That forced Mauch to go to his bullpen once again, this time for his right-handed closer Donnie Moore. Moore was in the prime of his career and his repertoire included a good fastball to go along with a slider and forkball. He was one of the elite relief pitchers in baseball in the mid-'80s. Bringing him in was a no-brainer for Mauch. Not only was Moore the best he had in the bullpen, but he was again playing the percentages—this time right-handed pitcher versus right-handed hitter. Nobody could possibly question this decision.

The crowd certainly greeted the move enthusiastically, roaring their approval as Moore took the mound to face Hendu. There were now more cops in our dugout in anticipation of the surge of fans about to storm the field. The cops literally started forcing us down the dugout exit runway. So I was watching Hendu's at-bat seven steps below field level, looking through the legs of cops, trying to get a view of what was happening on the field. All the guys on the bench were doing the same. It was pure bedlam at Anaheim Stadium with the drama building by the second. Everyone in the stands was on their feet, cheering on Moore to get that final out.

After blowing two fastballs by Hendu, Moore and the Angels were now just one strike away from ending our season and going to the World Series. I looked over at the Angels dugout and could see the stoic and stern-looking Mauch, standing erect with his arms crossed and sporting his marine haircut, sort of uncharacteristically yucking it up with Reggie Jackson. But who could blame him? Despite his skills as a great strategist, Mauch had managed 25 years by that point without ever taking one of his clubs to the World Series. He had lived the last 22 years of his life dealing with the fallout of a late-season collapse in 1964 in which his Philadelphia Phillies team had blown a 6½-game lead with just 12 games left in the season, finishing one game behind the St. Louis Cardinals. I truly believe the bitter disappointment of that '64 season never left him. But now, he was just a strike away from having his life-long dream of going to the World Series become a reality. He had a right to show a little levity.

After working the count to 2-2, Hendu stayed alive by fouling a ball straight back—a sign that he was starting to time Moore's pitches better. While I knew we were hanging on by a thread, I was positive that something great could happen. And then it did.

Hendu would smoke a Moore forkball out over the plate six rows into the left-field bleachers for a home run to give us a 6–5 lead! But I never saw it happen. Between the legs of the officers, all I could see was Hendu's feet leave the ground and then, suddenly, there was dead silence in the ballpark. That's how I knew something great had happened for us. As Hendu watched the ball sail over the fence, he leaped high in the air a couple of times—twisting and contorting his body around in pure jubilation. I wouldn't see the whole home run until after the game. We all came pouring out of the dugout to congratulate him, just going wild at this crazy turn of events. It was nothing less than astonishing.

By the time Hendu reached home plate, most of the cops were out of our dugout, while the few that remained were sitting on the bench. The crowd, ready to burst just a moment earlier, was now silent in stunned disbelief.

I've seen some big home runs in my life, but for me, Hendu's was the greatest, most important, and most dramatic of them all. And that's taking nothing away from Bernie Carbo's or Carlton Fisk's home runs in the '75 World Series, or even Joe Carter's that won the World Series for the Blue Jays in '93. Hendu's was the greatest because we were down three games to one and just one strike away from elimination. None of the other three would have ended a game or a series had an out been made by the hitter. As for how the three Red Sox home runs rank in the annals of club history, Fisk's may have been the most celebrated, but I would put Carbo's ahead of Carlton's because we were down three runs when Bernie hit his and it brought the team back from the dead; I will always say that Hendu's was the most important of all.

It's hard to put into words how we went from the lowest of lows and the indignation of being forced down a runway and not being able to see the at-bat of a teammate to then seconds later experiencing the highest of highs watching Hendu rounding the bases after hitting that home run. It was an emotional roller coaster unlike any other I had ever experienced before in baseball. It was almost unimaginable.

Back in the dugout, I wrapped both of my arms around Hendu from behind him as I prepared to get ready to go back into the field. Naturally, he had that thousand-watt, gap-toothed smile just glued to his face. I couldn't have been more thrilled for him—or us. And it was sweet redemption for Hendu. Earlier in the game, he deflected a ball hit by Bobby Grich off his glove that went over the fence for a two-run homer, giving the Angels a 3–2 lead. He felt awful about it, but it actually would have been a spectacular catch had he made it. But none of that mattered anymore. It would be nothing but a footnote after his dramatic home run.

After Moore retired Eddie Romero on a flyball to right field to end the top of the ninth, a chorus of boos rained down on him from the crowd. We will never know for sure how intensely the impact of Hendu's home run and the fallout from it might have affected Moore. But less than three years later and with his career now over, he tragically shot his wife three times (she survived) and then put a gun to his head and committed suicide. I cannot imagine the torment Moore lived with to reach that point of hopelessness, anguish, and despair.

In retrospect, I also can't fathom what Mauch was thinking after that home run and how he later handled it. I would pay a lot of money to know what was going on in his mind. After all his years in baseball, and all the heartbreak he experienced as a manager, to fail to reach his first World Series needing just one more strike must have been agonizing for him.

As devastating as it must have been for Moore, Mauch, and the Angels, there was still the bottom of the ninth to be played. And as it played out, the Angels would tie the game on a one-out RBI single by Rob Wilfong, sending the game into extra innings. The drama of this game was off the-charts. It was like a 15-round heavyweight fight.

The game would remain tied until the top of the 11th, when we would break through against Moore, who was still in the game despite the pain of giving up the Hendu home run and having it no longer be a save situation. Baylor, as he so often had happen throughout his career, was hit by a pitch to start the inning. I followed with a single up the middle to give us runners on first and second and nobody out. Again, the crowd started vehemently booing Moore. When Angels pitching coach Marcel Lachemann came out to the mound to check on Moore, the crowd derisively cheered, thinking he might get pulled, which did nothing to help Donnie's confidence. Then the fans booed again when Lachemann left him in the game. Geddy would come up next and bunted the ball poorly straight up into the air toward third. If DeCinces caught it, it may have been a double play. But instead, it dropped at his feet and his throw to first pulled Bobby Grich off the bag to load the bases—a most fortunate break for us. That set the stage for another showdown between Moore and Hendu and, on the first pitch, Dave sent a fly ball deep enough to centerfield for Baylor to tag up and come home to give us a 7–6 lead.

We would take that one-run edge into the bottom of the 11th with Calvin Schiraldi on the hill in relief. We picked up Calvin as part of the Bobby Ojeda trade with the Mets prior to the season. Schiraldi had pitched outstandingly well out of the bullpen after getting called up in the second half of the season, picking up nine saves to go along with a 1.41 ERA and had better than a strikeout per inning ratio. But he was coming off a rough outing just the night before when he couldn't save a great performance by Clemens, hitting Brian Downing with a pitch with two outs in the ninth to force in the tying run. Calvin would then pick up the loss in the bottom of the eleventh after surrendering an RBI single to Grich. It was a brutal loss for us, especially after Clemens entered the ninth with a three-run lead and we couldn't hold it.

But Schiraldi turned the page and was back to being the pitcher we saw during the regular season, striking out Wilfong and Dick Schofield and getting Downing to pop out in foul territory to defensive replacement Dave Stapleton at first base. *It was over!* We celebrated like we had won the pennant. And in a sense, we had. After a victory like that and knowing the next two games would be back home at Fenway, we knew this was a seismic shift of momentum in our favor. And we really came together in Game 5 and learned, as a unit, to take things one pitch at a time.

We easily won the next two games in Boston by scores of 10–4 and 8–1, respectively. Appropriately enough, the only two Red Sox from our '75 pennant-winning club—Rice and me—provided the power in the deciding game with home runs. But I think it was even more special for Jimmy, since he hadn't gotten to play in the '75 postseason because of his injury. So to see him hit a three-run homer to put Game 7 away was pretty awesome.

After 11 years, the Red Sox were World Series–bound once again. As a team, we were physically banged up and mentally exhausted, but the pure euphoria of returning to the Fall Classic was a magical thing—and a great healer. It was such a wonderful time. It still gives me goosebumps just thinking about it. And we couldn't wait to take on the favored Mets and prove the "experts" wrong.

CHAPTER 17

ECSTASY AND AGONY

WE DIDN'T CARE who we played in the '86 World Series, but the fans, the media, and NBC Sports were downright ecstatic about the matchup. Our mission was just to win. But there was no ignoring the hype of a rare New York–Boston World Series matchup, the first of its kind since way back in 1912 when Red Sox pitcher Smoky Joe Wood defeated the Giants three times—including the final game clincher over Christy Mathewson.

Now, 74 years later, it was the Red Sox taking on the Mets, winners of 108 regular season games, but a club, like us, that needed a stunning comeback in their own playoff series—in their case, against the Houston Astros—to set up what had all the elements to be a classic World Series. Still, because of their dominance over the National League during the regular season, the Mets were big favorites—much like how the Reds were favored over us in '75—to win the World Series.

But after the first two games of the series at Shea Stadium, I don't think those who picked the Mets were feeling so great about their prediction. Ever since our remarkable comeback in Game 5 of the ALCS, we were looser than at any time all season. It was like we were playing with house money.

In the opening game, our starter, Bruce Hurst, and the Mets' Ron Darling were magnificent, putting up zeros until we finally broke through in the top of the seventh. Rice led off with a walk and then advanced to second on a wild pitch. One out later, Gedman hit a ground ball that went through the legs of Mets' second baseman Tim Teufel to allow Rice to score the only run we would need in our 1–0 victory. Hurst and his split-fingered fastball would throw 123 pitches before giving way to Schiraldi who picked up the save in the ninth. It was the first 1–0 shutout in the opening game of a World Series by Red Sox pitching since Babe Ruth accomplished the feat in 1918—the last time Boston won the Fall Classic. With all the chatter about the Curse of the Bambino—something I never believed in—it made for good copy for those who saw it as a good omen.

The second game was dubbed one of the greatest pitching matchups in World Series history. Clemens was coming off an incredible campaign in which he finished 24–4, the most regular season wins by a Red Sox pitcher since Mel Parnell in 1949, and would go on to win both the Cy Young Award and AL MVP. Roger would face Dwight Gooden who, a year earlier, had gone 24–4 with a 1.53 ERA in winning the NL Cy Young Award and who was still widely regarded as one of the best pitchers in baseball. He was also a hot pitcher who had a 1.06 ERA in the playoffs. But as they say, anything can happen in baseball, and the pitcher's duel everyone anticipated turned out to be a blowout 9–3 win for us.

Neither pitcher had their stuff that night, especially Gooden, yet it was still a close 4–2 game in the top of the fifth. After Rice led off with a single, I came up to the plate looking to extend the rally and give Roger some more breathing room. I had heard so much about Gooden, nicknamed "Dr. K" after having more strikeouts than any pitcher in baseball the previous two seasons. He featured a fastball in the high 90s to go along with a 12-6 curveball with a hard, downward, sweeping break so good that it was nicknamed "Lord Charles" by Mets' broadcaster Tim McCarver, as opposed to the more common "Uncle Charlie" moniker used for a curveball. I had a disciplined approach against Gooden. He could throw me all the curve balls he wanted, but unless there were two strikes, I wasn't going to swing at any of them. This way, especially if I was ahead in the count, I could look for a certain pitch—like his fastball. And if I was going to swing at his breaking ball, I knew I was going to have to be 100 percent sure I could hit it hard or else it wouldn't be good hitting. But on Gooden's very first pitch, he threw me what I was looking for—a fastball right down the middle—and I jumped all over it, crushing the ball onto the top of an awning covering the left-center-field bleachers to give us a commanding 6–2 lead. It was a gut punch to the Mets and Gooden was taken out of the game after finishing the inning.

Still, with a team as good as the Mets, we were determined not to let them off the mat, especially with the top of their order due to hit in the bottom of the fifth and Roger looking a little tired from all the innings he threw in the ALCS. So, when Lenny Dykstra led off their half by ripping a shot off Clemens toward the right-centerfield gap, as Henderson and I converged on it, I went into a slide to avoid him and made a back-handed, ice-cream-cone catch just before the ball hit the ground, taking some of the steam away from the Mets' hopes to rally back. After the next two hitters, Wally Backman and Keith Hernandez, reached base, Clemens' night was over. Despite the four-run lead, we weren't going to jeopardize the game by trying to have Roger finish the fifth inning to set himself up for a win. The move paid off, as Steve Crawford and Bob Stanley were terrific in relief, not allowing any earned runs the rest of the way.

Up two games to none, we had the Mets' backs against the wall, but we certainly weren't going to get cocky about it. That being said, we had all the momentum—so important in baseball—and felt great about having the chance of winning Boston's first World Series in 68 years back home before the Fenway Faithful.

There was no vacancy at the Evans' house in Lynnfield. We had my entire family—my parents, my brothers, and my sisters—staying with us and attending all three games at Fenway. It was their chance to see me play in a World Series and an opportunity to perhaps witness baseball history if we could close things out in Boston. But the Mets, showing why they were such a tough ball club, bounced back and won the first two games there to even the series.

In Game 3, it felt like it was over before it was even getting started. Dykstra, hitting in the leadoff spot, homered down the right-field line off Oil Can to give the Mets a quick 1–0 lead. Then the Mets tacked on three more runs that inning to take a 4–0 lead before we even came to bat. The Mets kept on hitting and would win the game 7–1 behind the pitching of our former teammate Bobby Ojeda.

The next night was more of the same with the Mets taking a 3–0 lead into the seventh. Trying to hold the Mets right there so we could attempt a late-inning comeback, Dykstra, with Mookie Wilson on second, hit a ball over my head in right field toward the 380-foot sign. I raced back toward the fence and should have caught it easily, but when I jumped, my left hip hit the wall and prevented me from going any further. As a result, I couldn't get my arm fully extended above the fence, and the ball tipped off my glove and into the bullpen for a home run to give the Mets a 5–0 lead. The Mets would hold on to win Game 4 6–2. Losing that game was discouraging, because we knew that we couldn't close out the series in Boston and would have to return to New York.

But we liked our chances to retake the series lead with Hurst, our hottest pitcher down the stretch and throughout the post-season, going up against Gooden, whom we hit hard earlier in the series. And much like in Game 2, we hit the Mets' ace hard, knocking him out of the game in the fifth inning. Meanwhile, Bruce cruised to a complete-game, 4–2 victory to give us a three games to two lead in the series. We were now just one win away from giving Boston a World Series title.

Anytime we had Clemens on the mound, we knew we had an excellent chance to win. And Game 6 was no exception—especially with Roger pitching on five days' rest. He was a perfect 6–0 during his remarkable season when getting five days off between starts. So, while Clemens held the Mets hitless through the first four innings, we put two runs up on the board against Ojeda with my RBI double in the first inning and Barrett's run-scoring single in the second.

After the Mets scratched out a couple of runs to tie it in the fifth, I drove home another run on a ground out in the seventh to give us a 3–2 lead. Meanwhile, Clemens retired the Mets in order in the bottom of the inning and was still on top of his game, just dealing.

However, after Roger came back into the dugout and put his batting helmet on to hit in the top of the eighth, McNamara called him over to discuss whether to keep him in the game. Clemens had developed a small blister on the middle finger of his pitching hand but was pitching through it just fine. Nevertheless, according to both Roger and Marty, who was standing there with them both, McNamara made the decision to pull Clemens from the game and use Mike Greenwell to pinch hit for him. I wasn't a part of the conversation, but what I do know is that Roger was a gamer and it's hard to imagine him taking himself out of a game of that magnitude. Plus, he had his batting helmet on, ready to hit. McNamara would later contend that it was Roger who asked out of the game, though through numerous accounts of what happened, that didn't appear to be the case.

We would load the bases in that eighth inning, looking to put the game away, but we came up empty. The Mets, meanwhile, would tie the game in the bottom of the inning with a run off of Schiraldi. As a result, the move to remove Clemens from the game would loom large and be debated for years to come.

After neither club scored in the ninth, the game moved into extra innings. This set the stage for one of the most memorable— as well as the most examined and analyzed—innings in the history of the World Series.

Henderson continued his clutch hitting in the postseason by leading off the top of the tenth with a home run off Rick Aguilera to give us a 4–3 lead. After Hendu's dramatic home run against the Angels, if this latest one would have turned out to be the game-winner of the World Series, the city of Boston would have erected a statue of him in Quincy Market. But we weren't finished. With two outs, Boggs doubled, and Barrett drove him home to add an insurance run to give us a 5–3 edge. At this point, the crowd was silenced—completely taken out of the game. We were feeling really good about our prospects of finishing off the Mets that night.

We took the field in the bottom of the 10th just three outs away from a World Series title. I was familiar enough with Red Sox history to understand that this could be a moment in time that generations of their fans had dreamed about after decades of near misses. But we had to finish the job first.

Schiraldi was sent back out for his third inning of work and, even though he was throwing great, it was a concern of mine. While Calvin had been our closer and mowing down guys since mid-season, pitching a third inning out of the bullpen is a tall order for any pitcher. So, when it became apparent that McNamara was going to send Schiraldi back out there, I almost went over to him to suggest he bring in Bob Stanley instead. I had the kind of player-manager relationship with Mac where I could have done that. Stanley had been our best reliever in September and October, and I thought it would have been far better that he started the inning with a two-run lead instead of coming in later into a potential mess. If Mac had done that, I think it would have been a completely different situation than what later transpired. And that's not taking anything away from Schiraldi. But I just felt that he had done his job and, at that point, Stanley was the better option. If I could second-guess any move that McNamara made in that game, that was it.

To Schiraldi's credit, he started the inning very well, getting the first two batters—Wally Backman and Keith Hernandez—to both fly out. We were one out away. From my position in right field, I prayed to myself, giving thanks to God for that special moment. Then I looked out at the scoreboard in left field, and for a brief instant, it prematurely read, CONGRATULATIONS TO THE 1986 WORLD CHAMPION BOSTON RED SOX! before it was quickly taken down. I can see it like it was yesterday. On NBC, the Lite Beer Player of the Game was awarded to Barrett. Up in the press box, the writers' votes were already in for World Series MVP—it would be Hurst. Back in our clubhouse, NBC was setting up an interview platform in anticipation of our victory. Cellophane had been draped over our lockers to protect our clothes from the spraying of celebratory champagne. And I heard that one of our guys had already opened one of those bottles of champagne. I'm not superstitious, but that's something you just *don't* do. We still needed one more out. One more, as it turned out, *highly elusive* out.

Schiraldi would get ahead of the next batter, Gary Carter, with a strike before surrendering a 2-1 line drive single to left field. *No big deal*, I thought. Kevin Mitchell would be next up, pinch-hitting for Aguilera. Again, Calvin got ahead in the count with a first pitch strike before Mitchell served a single into center field to put runners on first and second base. We were still in good shape, and I thought it was a smart move for Mac to send Bill Fischer, our pitching coach, to the mound to check on Schiraldi. But I couldn't help but wonder, with Stanley warmed up—standing and watching the developments from the bullpen—why he wasn't already in the game.

The meeting seemed to have a calming effect on Schiraldi, as his first pitch to Ray Knight was a perfect pitch—a blazing fastball on the outside corner and at the knees for a strike. Calvin came back with an identical pitch that Knight tapped slowly down the third base line that Boggs let roll foul. We were now just *one strike* away. Ahead 0-2, Schiraldi then threw Knight a fastball in on the hands that Ray was able to bloop into center field for an RBI single while putting runners on the corners and making it a 5–4 ballgame.

Calvin had gotten ahead of the last three batters, and none of them were hitting him particularly hard, but he just couldn't manage to put any of them away for that final out. Mac had seen enough and signaled for Stanley to enter the game. "Steamer" came up through the Red Sox system and had pitched for us at the big league level since 1977. Despite having a solid career as both a starter and reliever, he had a love-hate relationship with our fans, which was all the more reason why I thought how incredible it would be for him to be on the mound if he could get the final out of the World Series. I'm sure it was something he long dreamed about.

Stanley would face Mookie Wilson in what would be an epic 10-pitch at-bat. After getting Wilson to foul off the fourth pitch of the at-bat, we were again *one strike* away from winning the World Series. But Mookie fouled off the next two offerings to stay alive as the drama went up a notch with every pitch. What it also did was prolong the at-bat, and the more pitches a hitter sees, the greater the chance that something can go their way. And on the seventh pitch, with Gedman setting up outside, Stanley came so inside with a pitch that, had Mookie not been so agile, it most certainly would have hit him in the ribcage. Instead, the ball glanced off Geddy's outreached glove and went to the backstop, allowing Mitchell to cross the plate with the tying run. Geddy would later contend that there was no cross up between him and Stanley—that the pitch was supposed to be inside. Just not *that* far inside.

Shea Stadium was now a mad house. The fans were the loudest they had been all series. Obviously disappointed, I knew we had to shake it off and stay focused. Besides, the game was still tied. It wasn't over. Now with the count full, Mookie popped the next pitch up and Geddy gave chase, but it was just barely out of his reach and into the stands. Wilson would foul off yet another pitch—the ninth of the at-bat. I would later find out that prior to that pitch, Barrett noticed Knight, exuberant over the Mets tying the game, was way off second base. So, Marty called for a pick-off play, which he contends would have gotten Knight out easily to end the inning. Marty would say that Geddy gave the "five signal" for a pickoff at second, but Stanley delivered a fastball to the plate instead. With everything going on, Stanley was completely focused on the batter.

With Barrett still cheating toward second with the pickoff play still on before the next pitch, Buckner, wearing special high-top spikes designed to help his Achilles heel injuries that were affecting his range of motion, had to move over a couple of steps away from first to cover some of Marty's ground. That would prove ominous after Stanley again delivered to the plate and Mookie hit a slow roller up along the first base line. Buckner was able to move to his left just quickly enough to get in front of the ball, though he didn't have as much time as usual to set himself. And with Mookie, one of the fastest players in the game, everything had to go perfectly for Buckner to field the ball and quickly flip it to Stanley covering first base.

From my vantage point in right field, I could see it all unfold. It appeared that the switch-hitting Wilson, a step-and-a-half closer to first base hitting from the left side of the plate instead of the right side, was going to beat Stanley to the bag no matter what. And that's no fault of Stanley's—Mookie could just fly. But as it turned out, that wouldn't matter. The ball was bouncing and bouncing and then hit something, like a clod of dirt, and didn't bounce up again—staying low on Buckner. It then skipped under his glove, through his legs, and rolled into right field. Knight scored easily from second to give the Mets one of the greatest comebacks in baseball history and the Red Sox one of the most devastating defeats.

Over the years, people have asked me what I did with what would become a very valuable baseball after it rolled out to me. But I didn't even bother to pick it up because the game was over, so right field umpire Ed Montague retrieved it instead. At that moment, I was just trying to process how everything had just fallen apart for us. I felt that Game 6 and the world championship was ours. I don't know if anyone can understand the feeling of being in right field as a player, seeing with their own eyes a two-run lead with two outs and two strikes in the bottom of the 10th, and then watching it all unravel like it did. That precious moment I had right before the Mets' two-out rally started was just taken away. It remains surreal to me. It just doesn't seem like it happened. And to this day, I have not looked at the highlight film of that game. It's just too painful as an athlete. I like to think I'm over it, but I guess on some levels I'm not.

In the clubhouse after the game, much of the talk from the media was over Mac's decision to leave Buckner and his two injured ankles on the field for the 10th. After all, Mac often replaced Buck with Dave Stapleton late in games. But I thought it was just a ridiculous criticism. If Buck couldn't get in front of Mookie's groundball in time, you could say it was a bad move. But he did, and 99 percent of the time he fields that ball and gets the out. But in this case, even if Buck fields it cleanly, Wilson beats it out, the game is still tied, and if we get the next hitter out, we move on to an 11th inning. So, he didn't cost us the game or the World Series as so many people unfairly point out. And I would add that without Buckner and his 102 RBIs that season, we wouldn't have been in the World Series in the first place.

As Buck was unjustly blamed for the loss, he handled it all with grace, class, and dignity, answering each reporter's question about it. He took full responsibility, telling them that Mac asked him before the bottom of the 10th if he wanted to finish the game and he said he did. Mac correctly felt that Buck deserved to be on the field as a conquering hero if we won the World Series. Plus, Buck's Achilles tendons were feeling better that night than they had earlier in the series.

But it was still hard for Buck to stand up before the press like he did. If there's one regret I have about that night, it's that afterward, back at the team hotel, I didn't take the time to check in with Buck and console him, considering the magnitude of what had occurred. Everybody tried to blame him for something that wasn't his fault. If I could ever do that moment over again, I would have certainly done things differently.

It was a tough night for all of us and one of the lowest moments in my career and in Red Sox history. It's not something I've talked much about, nor should it be. But as a ballplayer, you need to have the ability to compartmentalize events and move on quickly. And as a team, we were like, *Okay, that was rough. But we've been through a lot this season and always battled back.* We weren't going to hang our heads. I knew we would be ready for Game 7.

———————

With a rainout giving us a day off between Games 6 and 7, we had an extra 24 hours to put our heartbreaking defeat behind us. What it also did was allow Mac to come back with Hurst to pitch the seventh game. Bruce had already beaten the Mets twice and allowed just two earned runs over 17 innings in the series. Still, it was a calculated risk, as Bruce would be pitching on just three days' rest. He would start in place of Oil Can, the scheduled starter, who would have pitched on his full five days' rest. After a rough first inning in Game 3, Can settled down to retire 18 of the next 19 Mets hitters he faced—proving he was more than capable of beating them if called upon. Boyd was grief-stricken over Mac's decision, but it was hard to argue with not using our hottest pitcher over the last month and a half in a do-or-die game like this one.

For us, Game 6 was a distant memory now. It was business as usual. We went into Game 7 exuding confidence and intensity, and there wasn't even a thought beyond the fact that we were going into a new game, a game we wanted desperately to win.

Darling was making his third start of the series and, despite his success against us in the first two games, the more a team sees an opposing pitcher in a short amount of time, the better it is for them. And to prove there was no hangover from our Game 6 collapse, we took it to Darling and the Mets in the top of the second inning when we put three runs on the board.

I got things started by jumping all over a full-count, knee-high fastball and sending it well beyond the left center-field fence for a home run to put us up 1–0. It was hit in almost the identical spot to the one I hit off Gooden in the second game and broke Darling's scoreless streak of 15 innings over us. Gedman would then follow me with a home run of his own, a long fly ball to right center field that glanced off the outstretched glove of Darryl Strawberry a foot over the wall to give us a 2–0 lead. We then had to work a little harder to get our third run. Hendu followed Gedman's home run with a walk, and then, after Hurst's sacrifice bunt moved him to second, Boggs singled to center to increase our lead to 3–0. Our approach against Darling at the start of that game was very professional. One inning at a time. One at-bat at a time. One pitch at a time. And it was paying off.

Meanwhile, Hurst picked up where he left off in his two previous starts in the series with more masterful pitching, blanking the Mets on just one hit through five innings. On the Mets' side, Darling's night was over in just the fourth inning and Sid Fernandez came in to pitch for them. Fernandez had won sixteen games and struck out 200 batters as a Mets' starter that season, but he didn't start in any of the World Series games. He would make his presence felt in this game, however, striking out four over 2⅓ innings through our half of the sixth to keep the score at 3–0.

This allowed the Mets time to battle back. After Hurst got the first out in the bottom of the sixth, the Mets would load the bases, and Keith Hernandez came through for them with a two-run single to cut our lead to 3–2 and put runners on the corners. Carter then followed by looping a short fly ball to me in right. I came charging in and made a diving catch, but the ball popped out of my glove as I hit the ground, making it a non-catch. But when I noticed Hernandez got a late break toward second—thinking I had caught the ball—I quickly got back on my feet and fired to Spike Owen at second to force him out—a rare 9-6 fielder's choice. However, on the play, Backman scored from third, and it was now a 3-3 ballgame. We were able to get out of the inning and keep the score tied when Rice ended the Mets' rally with a spectacular diving catch of a slicing line drive hit by Strawberry to short left field. Our entire season would now come down to three innings.

With Hurst out of the game after giving us every last ounce of energy he had, the Mets would score three runs off our bullpen in the seventh to take a 6–3 lead. But while the Mets and their delirious fans could taste a world championship at this point, I knew we still had a lot of fight in us, and the game was far from over. We had too much character and talent to give up.

Buckner and Rice both singled to start the top of the eighth and I doubled them home to cut the Mets' lead to 6–5. The two RBIs gave me a total of nine to tie Carter for the most in that World Series but would be small consolation if we didn't win. With nobody out and with me in scoring position at second base, we had an excellent chance to tie the game. The Mets went to the bullpen, replacing Roger McDowell with their left-handed closer Jesse Orosco, who had the nastiest stuff of any of their pitchers, to face Gedman. Richie would hit one of the hardest line drives I've ever seen, but it was right at their second baseman Backman, so I couldn't advance. A few feet in either direction and the ball goes into right field and we tie the game. Or if it's hit on the ground, I would have advanced to third base, giving the next hitter, Hendu, the chance to drive me in with just a fly ball. As it turned out, Hendu would strike out and Baylor would ground out to short to end the inning, stranding me at second. But we were back in the game and just needed our bullpen to keep things where they were to give us a chance in the ninth.

Unfortunately for us, that didn't happen. Strawberry, who had struggled throughout much of the series, led off the bottom of the eighth with a moonshot over my head and well beyond the right field wall to extend the Mets lead to 7–5. They would tack on another run from one of their unlikeliest sources when Orosco, with runners on first and second and one out, faked a bunt and bounced an RBI single up the middle to give the Mets an 8–5 edge.

Orosco would then set us down in order in the top of the ninth—ending it with a strikeout of Barrett, who had a World Series record-tying 13 hits for us—to win the series for the Mets.

Our Red Sox team that year was one of the best I ever played on, but in the end, the Mets simply outplayed us. Like in '75 against the Reds, we were the bridesmaids yet again. And being a bridesmaid isn't fun because people generally don't remember the team that loses a World Series. They only remember the guys who win. The only ones that truly remember the losing teams are their own fans. Yet, in both the '75 and '86 World Series, we came in as big underdogs and gave the Reds and Mets everything we had right down to the final inning. And that's something to take pride in.

Even though it's so much better to be on the winning side than the losing side, I truly look back fondly at '86 as a whole. We had a magical ride during the regular season, had a remarkable comeback in the ALCS, and came within one strike of being world champions. The wonderful memories outnumbered the bad ones by a long shot. It was such a special and meaningful season because we did it all. And in the immediate aftermath of that World Series, our fans felt the same way and gave us one of the largest victory parades and celebrations at Government Center in Boston that the city had ever seen. And even today, whenever one of us from that team returns to Fenway Park, we are treated like royalty by the organization and our fans. Boston fans respect the human spirit of giving it your all, doing all you can to win, and always hustling. They knew that's how we approached the game and that we cared as much as they did.

But I understand the disappointment, as well. The history of the Red Sox was such that, in the end, the team would always break your heart. Our '86 team joined the '75, '67, and '46 teams that all made it to the seventh game of the World Series only to come up short. Add to that fact that we led 3–0 in the seventh games in both '75 and '86 and didn't win either of them. I have never believed in luck, nor do I believe that our team history had anything to do with why we ultimately lost in '86, though I can understand why some superstitious fans might.

We had some outstanding performances in the '86 World Series that, while they didn't make losing easier to swallow, showed that we gave maximum effort. Hurst nearly won three games, Marty hit .433, Rice and Spike hit .300 or higher, and Hendu hit .400 with two home runs—including his huge one to put us ahead in the 10th inning of Game 6. And just like I did in the '75 World Series, I made a major contribution in this one with my two home runs, nine RBIs, .400 on-base percentage, and OPS of 1.015. I was at peak concentration throughout both of those World Series. I wish I could have bottled up that concentration level for the regular season, but I could only match it in situations when I generally represented the tying or winning run at the plate. The game had to be on the line. Being ahead or behind by 10 runs lowered my concentration level slightly because the game was out of hand and, at that point, your at-bats become more about you and your own batting statistics; and I was always more about winning than padding my stats for personal achievements. That stuff just wasn't important to me until the season was over and it was time to negotiate a contract. You had to compare your stats to others in those meetings. But there were guys that had what I would best describe as "aggressive concentration" at *all times*—a level of concentration that brought the best out of guys like Pete Rose and Boggs. If you want to call that being greedy as a hitter and wanting more, then I think that's a good greed, a healthy greed. I truly wish I had that elevation of concentration all the time instead of just in crucial game situations or in the World Series.

But even with what I accomplished personally in the '86 World Series, not winning it was the biggest regret of my entire career. It was far worse than losing in '75. I was just shy of 35 years old during the '86 series, and I knew time was getting short for me. The sting of that loss never left me. And I say that knowing full well how fortunate we were to make it that far with our stunning comeback over the Angels in the ALCS.

In fact, the way we lost the World Series was eerily similar to the way the Angels lost to us in the ALCS—both of us were one strike away from winning our respective series before losing them. And that fact was driven home to me during the off-season on a Nike-sponsored trip to Hawaii in which they invited some of the top major league players who made up their Nike team and their wives. I got to rub shoulders with guys like Mike Schmidt and Steve Carlton. Boggs and Buckner were there as well. Another player who attended was my friend Bob Boone, the great Angels catcher. So, I was standing around one of those days with Boone and three other players and Bob starts going on about Game 6 of the World Series. "I'm watching on TV," Boone says. "And I'm jumping up and down when that ball went under Buckner's glove, screaming at my TV and going, '*How does that feel?! How does that feel?!*'" And I understood at that very moment how, just like us, he went from the highest emotions you can possibly have to the lowest within a matter of seconds. What happened to us is what had happened to them. It wasn't that he was saying it in a bad way. He was saying it in a way like, *Now you know how I felt!* As much as it killed us to lose to the Mets, it killed them just as much to lose to us, especially the way that it happened.

Of course, in the annals of baseball history, the Mets' comeback in Game 6 and the excitement of Game 7 made it a phenomenal series for baseball. I had people come up to me in airports for years afterward and say things like, "What a great World Series. I was not a baseball fan, but I started watching baseball after that." I didn't understand it right away. I would often look at them with my head cocked and go, *Really? What a great World Series? Are you nuts? We lost.* But as a Mets fan or a fan who had no skin in the game, those last two games were terrific baseball. And when I could finally sit back as strictly the fan of the game that I am, I realized how great a World Series it really was. But for Red Sox fans, the team, the front office, and everyone else involved in our organization, I understand how gut-wrenching it was.

But what I still don't understand is the harsh treatment Buckner and Stanley received by some of the media and so-called Red Sox fans in the months and years following the World Series. Buck was a warrior who could barely walk during that entire World Series, but because of his infamous error, he had to deal with the cruel fallout from it for the rest of his life. As for Stanley, he was all heart and pitched 6⅓ innings over five World Series games with a perfect 0.00 ERA. But because of the wild pitch, he drew the ire of some fans, including one maniac who went to Bob's house where his two small children were playing outside, picked up one of their bikes, and threw it against a basketball pole. The fan then told the kids to tell their father he sucked. A real class act. Both Buck and Steamer deserved much better.

There are more important things in life than baseball. In the grand scheme of things, for as intense and emotional as it can become, it's still just a game. And because the family pain that Susan and I endured as parents was far more devastating than anything I ever faced on the field, I don't think anybody understands that more than me.

CHAPTER 18

THE HANGOVER

IT WAS THE BEST and worst of times for me as a professional baseball player as we fought to defend our American League championship in 1987. At the advanced baseball age of 35, I had the
best year I would ever have on the diamond with 34 home runs,
123 RBIs, and a batting average of .305—all career highs. I would
finish fourth in the MVP voting, win a Silver Slugger Award, make
my third All-Star Game appearance, and lead the league in walks
for the third time in my career. If I could step to the side and ask
myself, *Did I do everything I could to help us win?* the answer would
be "Yes." So, in that way, it was a most satisfying season.

But the team results, which is all I ever cared about, were
very disappointing. With the same core of players back from our
pennant-winning season, we would finish six games under .500,
in fifth place, and 20 games out in the AL East standings.

Right from the start of spring training, there was a media-in-
duced bad vibe. Fishing for stories during a traditionally slow news
period, they wouldn't let go of our World Series defeat, continuing
to stir the pot with what Buckner would call "stupid questions"
about his Game 6 error. They also wouldn't ease up on whether it
was Clemens who asked out of Game 6 or if McNamara removed
him, causing some dissension between the two. And on Stanley's

wild pitch, they took turns placing the blame on either Steamer or Gedman for it. It may have made for good copy—and controversy sells newspapers—but some of it was fracturing the team. There was little concern or sensitivity for our own emotions or the heart that those guys showed during that series.

We also had Clemens and Gedman hold out that spring over contract disputes—a big setback. Clemens walked out of training camp on March 6 when his contract negotiations with the Red Sox broke down, and he didn't rejoin the club until just two days before opening day. Rocket was a guy who had just won 24 games and won both the Cy Young and the MVP awards. I didn't quite understand the Red Sox negotiating tactics with him. Roger meant so much to the Red Sox and to baseball that Commissioner Peter Ueberroth actually intervened to assure Clemens that our ownership would honor a verbally agreed upon contract before it was signed so he could be in uniform for the start of the season. As it was, the contract was modest for the best pitcher in baseball—$2 million over 2 years—with the Red Sox saying they didn't want to go any higher for a third-year pitcher.

Meanwhile, Gedman, coming off back-to-back All-Star seasons, tested the free agent market after rejecting an offer from the Red Sox that winter. But there were no takers, which I found remarkable for a catcher of his ability. So, Geddy returned to us on May 1 and signed a new contract with the Red Sox the next day.

At the time, I kind of realized there was a power play taking place by the major league owners with the way both the Clemens and Gedman cases went. And my suspicions would be validated later that year when an arbitrator ruled that the owners had violated our collective bargaining agreement by conspiring to restrict player movement.

It was always a mystery to me how the owners got together and were able to talk in private about player contracts and the economics of baseball. Back then, much like today, you never heard exactly how much money a club made each year. There were always ways of hiding revenue streams and keeping them secret so nobody could figure out what the clubs were actually making.

Geddy, along with other players, had been impacted by what was later ruled to be collusion by the owners. But the media and the fans didn't view Richie as the victim he was, and Geddy—a kind and sensitive man whom I held in high esteem not only as a teammate but as a human being—took the backlash of being seen as a greedy ballplayer hard. Plus, he was a local guy from Worcester. He never wanted to leave the Red Sox; he just wanted to be sure he was getting paid what he deserved by testing the market. The experience he endured would have an adverse effect on his play, and he could never again approach the numbers he put up before testing the free agency market.

Another development that spring was McNamara wanting me to start working out at first base a little bit. It raised a few eyebrows, including Buckner's. And Buck knew just how to show me I was infringing on his space. He took my first baseman's glove, put it in the clubhouse sink, and filled it up with water. The glove went into the sink weighing about eight ounces and came out weighing about eight *pounds*! It took a week for it to dry out. It was something that a brother might do, which is the kind of relationship we had with one another. It was just so Buck. But while it was done in fun, I felt it was kind of like when someone says they're half-kidding about something but they're half-serious too. We were great friends, but first base was still, after all, his livelihood.

We got off to a lousy start in '87 and never recovered from it. Half of our lineup was hitting under .250 for the season as late as June, Oil Can was injured, and Schiraldi was struggling out of the bullpen. And in the second half of the season, we began to release and trade away players so critical to our success the year before. Buckner was first, released in July. Then on September 1, less than a year after their memorable home runs in Game 5 of the ALCS against the Angels, Baylor and Henderson were traded for players to be named later. Our front office had just imploded the nucleus of our club. And why they chose to move those three guys I will never know. Their character and skills meant so much to completing the puzzle of our championship team. And to receive almost nothing in return was unfathomable to me.

As it turned out, the three would find continued success elsewhere. Buckner would hit .306 the second half of the season with the Angels. Baylor would join the Minnesota Twins and help them win the World Series that October. Henderson would end up in Oakland the next season, become an All-Star, and win three pennants and a world championship there.

Our chaotic season finished with a whimper. We knew more changes were on the way.

CHAPTER 19

EQUAL TIME

OUR WORLD STOPPED ONCE AGAIN. We had been through dozens of surgeries with the boys by March 1988, but when Justin—still just an 11-year-old boy—had to undergo a 12-hour surgery at UMass Medical Center in Worcester to remove a tumor that sat at the base of his brain and the top of his spine, we knew how life-threatening it was. I came up from spring training to be there for my son and the rest of the family. We prayed hard—something we take very seriously—and braced ourselves for the worst. We almost lost him on the table.

We thanked God when our prayers were answered. Justin had survived, and he came out of it the same sweet and happy boy he had always been. He would be out of school for a year, and we had to have a teacher come to our Lynnfield home to work with him, but he never complained—he was always content to press forward with his challenging life wherever it led him.

Justin had a pleasant and caring nature about him that continues to inspire me to this day. Before that most serious surgery and in the years after, he would come to work with me. While I prepared for that day's game, he went across Jersey Street (then Yawkey Way) from Fenway Park to Twins Souvenirs. But he didn't go there to shop. He went there to help out. Eddie Miller was running the place and, at first, he would let Justin do stuff like stocking shelves. But after a couple of months, Justin wanted to expand his role. So, when someone would walk into the store, Justin would try to sell them souvenirs. Eddie would tell me, "Justin's the best salesman I have, but he's so enthusiastic about it that he starts *giving* things away!" He'd go to customers, "You need this, too, and that, too." Justin had such a kind heart that he didn't really think about the monetary part of it. He just didn't want anyone to leave empty-handed whether they paid for something or not.

Actually, both of my boys were entrepreneurs from a young age. I wouldn't find this out until years later, but when I would bring them both with me to Fenway Park, I would give them each five bucks to get something to eat at a nearby McDonald's on Brookline Avenue. Well, a clubhouse guy told me how the boys would routinely pick up a couple of baseballs during batting practice, take them into the clubhouse, get somebody like Clemens to sign them, and go outside the park and sell them on the street for $20 each. I guess I wasn't giving them enough money, so they sold autographed balls to "survive" and upgrade to sausage sandwiches or whatever else the street vendors were peddling.

Looking back, not having knowledge of what the boys were up to at Fenway doesn't really surprise me. I was just so into myself at the ballpark that I didn't always pay attention to what was going on around me. There was one time after I had a particularly bad game, I just kept asking myself repeatedly, *What the heck are you doing? What the heck are you doing?* And I got in my car and drove home. There was just one problem. I got a call at home from Eddie Miller, and he said, "Dewey, you forget something?" Now, Eddie was a crazy, funny guy who would come into our clubhouse and just hammer on us, saying things like, 'What are you now? Oh-for-your-last-90?' In no mood for games, I said, 'What, Eddie?' And he said, 'What about your son Tim?' In a slight panic, I said, *"What?!"* I went and looked in Timothy's room and he wasn't in bed. I got back on the phone and said, "You've got to be kidding me." Timothy, being headstrong, gets on the line and tells me, "I'm going to walk home." He was actually going to start walking from Fenway Park, get on I-93 North at Storrow Drive, and take Route 128 back to Lynnfield—a 19-mile journey home. Thankfully, Eddie ended up bringing Timothy home, but I never heard the end of it.

But that's how intense I would sometimes get with what I was doing. And once the game's over, I'd begin thinking about the next night's pitcher. *What did he do against me last time? How did they play me in the last game?* So, things were constantly spinning in my head. But leaving Timothy at Fenway was easily one of the major screw-ups I ever had with one of my kids.

––––––––––

For as difficult and heart-wrenching as it was to always be in hospitals, in doctor's offices, and getting the boys tested as often as we did, we continued to count our blessings that Kirstin was healthy, had never contracted NF, and didn't have any learning disabilities. It was just so nice to have a child who didn't have any issues like the boys had. As a result, she received the best of what Susan and I had to give, which probably wasn't as much as she needed. But we did as much as we could under the circumstances.

Kirstin felt very badly about her brothers' plight, but she still felt left out and jealous over all the attention we gave the boys. Timothy, by this time a 15-year-old, wasn't afraid to challenge Kirstin on this point, one time telling her point blank, "Do you want to trade places? You're beautiful. You have everything. You don't have any learning problems. Do you want to trade places with me?"

Sensitive to Kirstin's needs, and to give the boys individualized attention as well, we introduced a unique way of having dinner with the kids that we learned from other people in a similar situation. Whenever we could, Susan and I started having dinner with just one child at a time in our dining room. There were just three chairs and place settings for mom and dad—and either Kirstin, Justin, or Timothy. It would allow one of them time alone with us, while the other two would get their meal and move to another room. Each child's time with us would come in a rotating schedule. That systematic approach worked well for us—and gave Kirstin a more equitable share of our time.

I also enjoyed taking Kirstin with me on road trips. I would take her shopping and then go to the ballpark as late as I could possibly go. When it was time for me to leave, I would tell her to stay in our hotel room and to not open the door for anybody. Whenever possible, one of my teammates' wives would watch her. And then when it was time for her to go to the game, Debbie Clemens—Rocket's wife—would often meet her in the hotel lobby and bring her along with her. After games, if we played in New York, we'd grab a cab from Yankee Stadium and go to dinner at places like The Four Seasons and Gallaghers Steakhouse. We would stay out until after midnight and walk back to the hotel together under the bright lights of the city. If Kirstin joined me in Anaheim, we would go to Disneyland on an off day. Kirstin loved it all. And I treasured every moment I had with her, trying my best to make her feel special.

I would take Tim and Justin separately on road trips, as well. I did all I could to make sure I spent as much equal time with my three children as possible. But I know it wasn't always enough. It was only after Susan and I became grandparents did we fully realize what could have been had there not been serious illness with the boys. It showed us the kind of parents we could have been. Instead, we were constantly running around with no immediate family, cousins, aunts, or uncles to help us out. At least I had the ballpark, a place where I could shut down and hide myself for a few hours before coming home and facing the elephant in the room. But Susan had no outlet. When Justin had the surgery to remove the tumor from his brain and spine that year, I was only up from spring training for 24 hours before flying back down to Winter Haven. So, Susan was left overwhelmed with overseeing Justin's recovery while taking care of the two other children. Her body mass was low, and she was just utterly depleted. At one point, she laid her head against a wall and kept repeating to herself, "God, I can't do it. I can't do this anymore." And God spoke to her, saying, "Use the gift I gave you." To which Susan asked, "Really? What's that?" And He replied, "Humor. Humor."

Now, I can vouch for Susan that, despite our travails, she has an outstanding sense of humor. And it's that trait of hers that has helped get us through some of the most difficult times in our lives. But it's also helped us through some of life's lighter moments as well. One of my favorite Susan stories occurred at a Red Sox season ticket holders' event in the late '80s. We were standing around with this small group of high society women we met there, and for the next 10 minutes each of them just went on and on, bragging about how wonderful and perfect their children were. One told us their kids were attending boarding school at Choate, another had one going to Harvard, and so on. It seemed like they never had a single issue with any of their kids their entire lives. After what seemed like an eternity, Susan finally goes to them, "You know, I'm just happy when I go to the post office, I don't see my kids' faces on the wall. Or when I watch *America's Most Wanted*, they're not on the show. That's a *good* day!" Appearing horrified, the women dressed in flowery dresses and pearls—oblivious to Susan's wit—just kind of went, "Oh my," and then turned around and walked away.

It's funny—Susan and I were never invited back to that event again. I can't imagine why!

CHAPTER 20

MORGAN MAGIC, TWO MORE TITLES, AND THE END OF AN ERA

AFTER COMING OFF SUCH A DISAPPOINTING SEASON, our club had a new look on Opening Day 1988. We promoted Brady Anderson from AAA to start in centerfield, inserted Sam Horn into the designated hitter role, moved Mike Greenwell from left to right field and, in an effort to solve our bullpen woes, traded for future Hall of Famer Lee Smith as our new closer.

Oh, and we had a new first baseman—*me!*

With Buckner gone and the idea of having Greenwell play in right field, Mac experimented with playing me at first base. Initially, I *loved* it. That's because, for the first time in my 17 years in the big leagues, I was able to go to the meetings on the mound when the pitching coach or manager came out. I couldn't wait to hear the words of wisdom that would be given to the pitchers. Standing in right field while the mound visits took place always left me wondering what the heck was being said. So, the first time I played first base, pitching coach Bill Fischer, a true character who everybody loved, came out to the mound with his head down, looked straight at the chest of the pitcher—never looking up—pointed toward the flagpole, and in his funny kind of voice said, "Mac sent me out here. He said if you don't start throwing strikes, he's going to the bullpen." And then Fish just turned around and walked back to the dugout.

I thought to myself, *What?! What was that?! That's the gathering of the minds I've been wondering about all these years?!* I was so disappointed with what I had just heard—or *not* heard. All those years after a pitching coach went out there, and the pitcher started throwing strikes, I assumed the coach had picked up on something he was doing mechanically wrong and gave him some sort of sage advice. But it was nothing of the kind. It was almost like that scene in *Bull Durham* when "Nuke" LaLoosh was wild, and the pitching coach came out for a mound visit and said how candlesticks made a nice wedding gift but said nothing to help out poor Nuke.

I'll also never forget the first ground ball that came my way. I was holding a runner on first, then got off the bag and into my fielding position as soon as the pitcher threw the ball. It was hit to my left, I caught it, stepped on the first-base bag, and then threw a perfect strike to Spike at short for a double play. I thought, *Wow, I like this!*

But three innings later, I was again holding a runner on first base when a ball got hit to my right. I fielded it and turned to throw to Spike—leading him toward the second base bag. But I missed him by 10 feet, throwing it into left field instead.

After that, I was never the same. My throws kind of shrunk up. I didn't want to throw the ball anymore from first base. I even had trouble throwing it back to the pitcher—I was sort of guiding it back and telling them to "Pick it, pick it, pick it." Hurst loved to imitate me saying that. But it was a real problem. I had developed something like the yips that pitcher Steve Blass suffered from in the prime of his career. Blass had perfect command of his pitches warming up in the bullpen, but once he came into a game, he suddenly lost his control. It was the same with me. During infield practice, my throws were right on the money all the time. But throwing during games just got to me.

I couldn't figure out how I had become so insecure throwing a baseball in the infield. As a right fielder, I could throw the ball 300 feet right on target. But I came to understand that it's a completely different throw from the outfield, as you get to gather your legs into position and drive toward your target. Your footwork is totally different from an infielder's.

After a while, teams took notice that I didn't have the footwork or mechanics of a first baseman and tried to take advantage of it by bunting the ball toward me. They knew I would have issues throwing the ball around the infield.

I ended up starting 61games at first that season—never to return. But I mostly enjoyed the experience, and it helped me have the good year I would have at the plate—.293, 21 home runs, 111 RBIs—because it kept me strong. Right field takes a bigger toll on a player than first base. But I was more than happy to return to my old stomping grounds when Mac inserted Todd Benzinger into the first-base role and moved Greenwell back to left. My arm wasn't initially as strong or in shape as I was used to, but once I stretched out those muscles and got my legs underneath me again, I was fine.

With the new look to our ball club, we stormed out of the gates, finishing April at 14–6—one game out of first place. But then a rough month of May, an average June, and a bad start to July contributed to just a 43–42 mark—nine games back at the All-Star break.

What it also did was prompt the firing of McNamara. I always had a good working relationship with Mac, and we had a mutual respect for one another. Plus, he came as close as you can get to becoming a world-champion manager. But like our former Red Sox skipper, Darrell Johnson, Mac also had a drinking problem and, like Johnson, it was likely a contributing factor to his dismissal.

Joe Morgan, our third-base coach, took over the reins, and "Morgan Magic" was born. We would remarkably win our first 12 games in a row and 19 of the first 20 under him to move into a first-place tie in the AL East with the Tigers on August 3. It was an incredible run, only to be outdone 10 days later when, on August 13, we set a major league record after winning our 24th straight home game.

There was plenty of drama during that magnificent run, but perhaps none more than what occurred just seven games into Morgan's tenure on July 20 before a sellout crowd at Fenway. We held a tight 5–4 lead into the bottom of the eighth over the Minnesota Twins when Ellis Burks led off with a walk. That's when Morgan, looking to pick up an insurance run late in the game, made the eyebrow-raising bold move of pinch-hitting the still-dangerous Rice with Spike Owen. Morgan's strategy was to move Burks into scoring position with a sacrifice bunt and, since Rice—one of the great sluggers of his era—didn't have much experience bunting, made the move to have Spike do it. But being pinch-hit for was an embarrassment for a future Hall of Famer with Jimmy's sense of pride and he took out his rage on Morgan, shouting at him, grabbing him by the shoulders, and forcing him down the dugout runway. Some of our guys had to intervene to diffuse the situation. After Joe returned to the dugout, he kept shouting, "I'm the manager! I'm the manager!" for all of us to hear. For his actions, Rice would get a three-game suspension from the club.

I didn't agree with Morgan's decision at all. It just wasn't right to pinch-hit for Jimmy there. The guy plays for you every day and you've got to show loyalty to a player like him. If Joe was trying to make a point about being in charge with the move, I didn't get it. We knew he was in charge. And even though Jimmy was nearing the end of his career, he was still a threat to break a game like that one wide open. You just never pinch-hit for a Jim Rice—*period*.

As it turned out, Owen would successfully move Burks to second, but we wouldn't score and the Twins would tie it up in the top of the ninth on a Kirby Puckett sacrifice fly off Lee Smith. The Twins would then take a 7–5 lead in the top of the 10th, threatening to end our winning streak at six games. But in the bottom of the 10th, Benzinger hit a dramatic three-run walk-off home run to give us a stunning 9–7 victory to keep the streak alive.

In just the two months since Joe became manager, we went from being nine games back to sitting in first place on September 13 with a 4½-game lead. Morgan and his "magic" were the toast of the town. At first, I found Joe hard to get to know. It took me time to figure out what he was thinking and how he managed. But once I watched the way he managed for a while, I figured out that he let his players do their thing and didn't interfere with their style of play. That's when I really began to respect him as a manager.

There would be times where he would come up to Marty and me and ask, "You guys want to hit-and-run?" This was really kind of neat because, since it was put on us, it made it almost impossible for the other team to pick up our signs. So, when Marty was on base and I was at the plate, we used our own signs like me pulling on my belt for a hit-and-run and him pushing his helmet down to acknowledge it. It put the game more in our hands than Morgan's. With Joe, it was never really about him—it was about the players.

He was a simple manager—and I mean that in the best of ways. We had a good relationship and I really enjoyed playing for him.

On September 15, we opened a critical four-game series at Fenway against the second-place Yankees. After they beat our ace Clemens in the first game to cut our lead over them to 3½ games, the storyline in the press was about history repeating itself to when the Yankees swept a four-game series in September of '78—dubbed the "Boston Massacre"—to erase a four-game Red Sox lead. But we didn't let that happen, winning the next three games to take a season-high six-game lead in the division.

The difference between that '88 Red Sox team and some of the others that lost leads late in the season was how we came together and played as a unit at the perfect time. We didn't have all that much talent—certainly not as much as the '78 team. But the element of team play really peaked for us to play as well as we did to take three out of four from the Yankees in that series. We didn't make any mental errors and just played tremendous baseball.

Hitting from the third spot in the lineup, I batted .385 with two home runs and 5 RBIs for the four games. I was thrilled to contribute the way I did. I thrived on playing at the point in the season when every game meant so much. And this series was no different.

In the bottom of the eighth inning of the pivotal third game of the series, I hit a go-ahead home run over the Green Monster en route to our 3–1 victory. It was, not surprisingly, a Saturday afternoon game that Hurst was pitching in. I had a knack for hitting weekend afternoon home runs with Hurst as the fortunate recipient. And I liked playing in the sunshine because you could see the entire ball better. During night games, you don't see the whole ball coming in—only one-third or, at best, two-thirds of it from where the lights shine down on it.

I would hit another home run the next afternoon—a two-run shot—to give us a commanding 7–1 lead in just the second inning. We would cruise to a 9–4 victory to put the Yankees away and position ourselves for the division title that we would clinch less than two weeks later.

While I never sought publicity, I frankly enjoyed seeing myself on the cover of the following week's *Sports Illustrated*. Under the heading of, "Sock, Sock, Sox!," it showed me following through on one of my home runs during the Yankees' series. But what made it most meaningful to me was how the cover story was about how we sent the Yankees packing and took control of the AL East race. And the fact the cover story fell on Susan's birthday was a bonus!

We finished the season with 89 wins in a division race that saw five clubs with 85 or more victories. It was one of the tightest divisional races of all time. The Yankees, for example, would finish in fifth place—only 3½ games out.

But it didn't matter. For the second time in three years, we were back in the postseason with another chance to capture a world championship. We would first have to face the juggernaut Oakland A's—winners of 104 games—in the ALCS. They were a club that steamrolled over the American League that year, including a 9–3 record against us. We knew it would be a difficult assignment.

———————

Despite our league-leading .283 team batting average, 813 runs scored, and 18-win seasons from Clemens and Hurst, the A's ran through us like we were nothing, sweeping us in four straight games. They were simply a much better team than we were without any weaknesses. They featured the power of Jose Canseco, Mark

McGwire, and Dave Henderson and the supreme starting pitching of Dave Stewart and Bob Welch.

But what really set them apart was their closer—my old friend Dennis Eckersley. Eck was simply flawless during that period, saving a major league–leading 45 games in '88, just one short of the all-time record at that time. And in this ALCS, he saved all four games for the A's.

In Game 1, with the A's leading 2–1 in the eighth, I led off against Eck and stood over the top of the plate—just *daring* him to hit me so I could reach base. My feet were on the white line on the inside of the batter's box and his first pitch was a fastball on the outside corner of the plate—right on the black. I'm thinking, *You've got to be kidding me.* His control, with his unique windup and knee kick, was incredible. He could put a pitch anywhere, on any corner, at any level—low, mid, or high. The only other pitcher I ever saw with control like Eck's was Catfish Hunter. As a closer, Eck would only have to throw six to nine pitches an inning for a save. That's because he only threw strikes and the batter had to go up there swinging. He was that great as a closer. And unlike many relievers, he didn't throw all that hard. He just made perfect pitches. I don't know any other way to describe him other than an artist out there. He even referred to his pitching as "painting"—and it certainly was. So, with the count 0-and-1, and knowing he was going to come right at me, I swung at the next two pitches—both perfect fastballs on the inside corner black— and struck out. Eck was unhittable.

Aside from their outstanding starting and relief pitching, the A's outhomered us 7–2—including three from Canseco—and would move on to the World Series. It was a tough way to end the season. And nobody took it harder than Hurst. Bruce pitched very well in both games he pitched, including the final contest of the series, but I believe he was so frustrated we got swept that, after our Game 4 loss in Oakland, he walked off our Boston-bound flight before take-off. Some of it may have also had to do with his onerous contract negotiations with the Red Sox and impending free agency. Knowing him as well as I do and how good a person he is, there must have been a lot of hurt in him. So, I can't say I blame him or that it was wrong of him to leave the team flight. I think the whole situation just got to him. Plus, he lived in Utah at the time—a short flight from Oakland—which may have factored into his decision.

Two months later, Bruce would sign with the San Diego Padres—a huge loss to our ball club. Hurst was one of the greatest left-handers Boston ever had and would later be inducted into the Red Sox Hall of Fame. His absence would be missed on the mound and in the clubhouse.

The '89 season got off to a bumpy start right from the very beginning of spring training. Advanced copies of *Penthouse Magazine* came out with an article revealing explicit details and allegations from Margo Adams about a longtime affair she had with Wade Boggs. Some of the content in the piece dragged the names of other guys on the club into it, creating a very difficult environment for the team.

I respected Wade for all his accomplishments on the field. He had tremendous eye-hand coordination, was an elite hitter, and worked extremely hard at improving his defense at third base. But this story just blindsided everyone and adversely affected the entire organization. We needed Wade to step up right away and say, "This is my fault. I created this situation." And then apologize to his teammates. He also needed to go to the press and tell them, "Hey, I created this." But initially, he didn't do either of those things. That was the issue that created a major rift between him and the club that would linger in the weeks ahead.

We started the season with four straight losses, with the scandal continuing to cause a distraction to the ball club. So, a couple of weeks into the season, I felt the need to do something about it. The club went to Cleveland for a quick two-game road trip, and I had a productive talk with Wade about the situation. And when we came back to Boston, he held a team meeting, said what needed to be said, and things finally moved forward from there.

We all make mistakes. And after this episode of his subsided, he turned his life around. I'm very proud of him. I can't imagine what Wade and his wife, Debbie, were going through back then. The media attention into their personal lives was unrelenting. But I will say one thing—Debbie stood by his side and supported him through those difficult days. She's a very strong gal. And they're still together today with two grown children and a bunch of grandchildren. Any marriage is a lot of work, but it's absolutely worth it.

The scandal set the tone for a rough year. Not even a trade with the Reds in the off-season for first baseman Nick Esasky, who would have a career year by belting 30 home runs with 108 RBIs, could pull us out of mediocrity. And it's a shame because it was one of those rare down seasons in the AL East. Despite winning just 83 games, we finished in third place and only six games out.

As for Boggs, despite all the distractions, he would become the first player in major league history to have at least 200 hits in seven straight seasons. His focus on hitting was remarkable.

I would also have a bit of drama as the end of the season approached. In my final at-bat of the last game of the campaign, I was sitting on 99 RBIs going into the bottom of the eighth inning. With one out, our shortstop Luis Rivera, hitting in front of me, singled in a run to give us a 4–1 lead over the Brewers. Luis knew the situation—I needed just one more RBI to reach a hundred for the season. So, he promptly stole second base to move into scoring position. And after I ripped an RBI single into centerfield, another 100-RBI season was in the books. It marked the third straight season in which I eclipsed 100 RBIs and the fourth time in my career. When Jeff Stone ran out to pinch-run for me at first base, I received a nice ovation from the Fenway crowd.

After a long, tough season, it was a nice moment.

The start of 1990 was a rocky period for me both personally and professionally. My father passed away that February, casting a dark cloud over my life as I prepared to leave for spring training. And then after reporting to camp in great shape, I suffered a stress fracture in the SI joint in my lower back during an early exhibition game when leaping toward the first-base bag. For a while, I couldn't play. And when I returned, after the SI joint naturally fused together on the right side, it would break again every time I slid into a base. When you break a bone, I don't care if it's a stress fracture or not, it's still a broken bone and it's extremely painful—especially in that area. And because of where it would fuse, I had very little flexibility on that side. But I powered through it with the help of codeine shots just to get through the day. Playing ball and trying to concentrate while being medicated, especially at 38 years old, would be difficult. But I managed as well as I could.

It would turn out to be such a tough year physically. Due to my injury, I wouldn't pick up a glove for the entire season and was relegated to the designated role in all 121 games I started. That was a big adjustment, as playing right field at a high level was always a source of great pride and was a significant part of my identity as a professional ballplayer. But even with being limited to DH, I made my presence felt, winning four games for the Red Sox with late-inning home runs.

And in what some considered our most pivotal series of the season—a three-game set against the Orioles beginning on June 22—I rose to the occasion. In the second game, I homered twice—including a two-out, two-run walk-off homer in the 10th inning against Gregg Olson, one of the top closers in the game. From what I was told, it was the first time anyone ever homered off his sharp-breaking, knee-buckling curveball. And in the third game, I hit a solo home run in the eighth inning to help us secure a sweep of the series. That got us on track, giving us the momentum to then sweep a four-game series from the Toronto Blue Jays. In just seven games, we went from a half game back to having a 3½-game lead in the AL East.

From there, we held on to first place for most of the season. But a 12–16 record in the month of September made things interesting, and the season came down to the final game on October 3 against the Chicago White Sox. With a one-game lead over the Blue Jays, all we needed to do was win the game and the division crown would be ours.

In that final game, we led 3–1 in the top of the ninth with our new closer Jeff Reardon on the mound. Reardon would retire the first two hitters before yielding a single to Sammy Sosa and then hitting Scott Fletcher with a pitch to put the tying runners on base. Standing next to Morgan in the dugout, he looked out toward our right fielder and then at me and said, "Is [Tom] Brunansky…." And before he could finish, I said, "He's got to play closer to the line." So, he moved Brunansky closer to the right field line with the left-handed hitting Ozzie Guillén at the plate. After Reardon got ahead in the count 0-2, and with the Fenway crowd on their feet and ready to go crazy, Guillén ripped a hard line drive toward the right field corner. With two outs and the runners on the move, if it dropped in, the game would be tied. But Brunansky hustled over and made a tremendous diving catch to end the game. If Tom hadn't been closer to the line, he never would have caught up with it. I'm not taking any credit for it, but I did tell Morgan to move Brunansky over. Most importantly, we had clinched the AL Eastern Division title for the third time in five years.

We would face the defending world champion Oakland A's, winners of 103 games, hoping for a better outcome than two years before. But we would again be swept in four games by the dynastic A's of that period, with Oakland outscoring us 20–4 in the series.

After the A's beat us handily in the first three games, things got ugly in the fourth and final game in Oakland. Clemens, our last hope to keep the series going, would get tossed in just the second inning for what home plate umpire Terry Cooney assumed were profanities directed at him by Roger over his balls-and-strikes calls. Rocket went nuts, claiming he was simply talking into his glove. Our guys on the bench were outraged, as well, with some of them tossing water coolers and litter onto the field. Our display was as much frustration over the series as it was over the terrible timing of Clemens' ejection. It was an awful way to end the season.

Little did I know it would also be the last time I would ever wear a Red Sox uniform as a player.

During the last week of the '90 season, knowing my contract was up at the end of the year and that the Red Sox had an option on me for the '91 campaign, I went to ownership with a request. If they weren't going to bring me back, I asked that they let me say goodbye. Nothing extravagant, no victory lap around Fenway, and no lengthy speeches. I was never one who really liked the microphone anyway. I just wanted something simple—an opportunity to thank the Red Sox organization and the fans for 19 memorable years with the club if this was the end. I thought maybe they would extend me that courtesy. But they didn't.

Three days after our final playoff game in Oakland, I was back at Fenway in my running suit, cleaning out my locker and grabbing a few things I wanted to take home. No one was around, not even the clubhouse attendant or equipment manager. As I was finishing up, Al Forester, who was the groundskeeper at Fenway for 53 years, tapped me on the shoulder and said, "Dewey, Lou Gorman wants to see you upstairs in his office." Perplexed this was coming from the groundskeeper, I said, "*What?!*" But Forester repeated the message—"Yeah, Lou Gorman wants to see you upstairs." I'm kind of thinking in my head, *What the heck?*

So, I went up to Gorman's office and the lights were off. Lou was sitting at his desk with a window behind him and Morgan was seated in the corner. Because of the brightness coming through the window, all I could see of Lou was his silhouette. I took a seat and Gorman leaned over his desk and said, "We've decided not to pick up your option." That was a tough thing to hear. And as I'm processing what was just said, I could hear Mrs. Yawkey and Haywood Sullivan down the hall laughing. I'm certainly not inferring they were laughing at me, but it was just kind of an unfortunate coincidence that as I'm being let go, they're yukking it up. I got up from my seat, thanked Lou and Joe, and walked out of the office stunned. I went home kind of shell-shocked. I didn't think it was handled right at all. Still, once the word got out, I did a few segments with different television stations—taking the high road.

Suddenly, I was a free agent. But one thing I didn't realize at the time was that the Red Sox still had rights to me. This meant that if any team wanted to sign me, they would have to give up compensation. After about a month, I called Haywood and asked him if he would grant me a few minutes to talk with him. When he did, I said, "Haywood, who is going to give up compensation for a 39-year-old player? *Who?* You guys hold that card. Would you please give me my unconditional release?" Thankfully, Haywood agreed, making me a free agent without any conditions.

Three teams were immediately interested in me—two from the National League and the Orioles. Even with my back issues, teams took note of how I hit .306 in the last six weeks of the '90 season—proving I could still play at a high level. And I was still just one year removed from a 20-homer, 100-RBI campaign. I decided to sign a one-year deal with Baltimore because, at that stage of my career, I didn't want to endure the learning curve of a different league. There was no interleague play in those days, so the National League would have been somewhat foreign to me. And a bonus to going with the Orioles was that Susan spent the first 11 years of her life in Middle River in Baltimore County and still had friends there. So, they were a good match for us. But the way it happened was not of my liking. It was really hard for me to move on.

I still wonder to this day why the Red Sox wouldn't give me a chance to say goodbye—even to the press. I just wanted a minute or so to express my thanks and gratitude to everyone for their support. If they had allowed that, I would have retired as a Red Sox player if they had asked me to. I know one thing for sure. The current Red Sox ownership would have handled it differently. They've done nothing but build up the current team and make it an attractive place to play. The Red Sox organization is one of the top two or three in all of baseball—right there with the Dodgers and Yankees. My release would have been handled in a far classier way today. After all, at the time of my release, I had played in more games in a Red Sox uniform than anyone except for Yaz. And my 379 home runs and 2,373 hits for the Red Sox both ranked fourth on their all-time list. I deserved a better sendoff.

I always assumed I would end my career with the Red Sox, but, sadly, it wasn't to be.

CHAPTER 21

THE LAST HURRAH

IN MY ERA, we played until they told you to go home two or three times. We played until they took the uniform away. And we played for the love of the game. Don't get me wrong, we loved the money, too. And while the money wasn't anything like what players get today, I truly don't hold it against them. The game is in a place where it can tolerate those lucrative salaries. And to be honest, I loved the era in which I played and wouldn't trade those experiences, people, and moments—from pitch to pitch, from play to play—for anything. I couldn't have been in a better profession at a better time.

Since age 17, the Red Sox had been the only organization I had ever known. But I wasn't ready for my career to end. With my last stop in Baltimore, I was determined to make the best of this new experience. And to the Orioles' credit, they welcomed me with open arms and made me feel wanted. The first thing they did was introduce me to everyone in the front office. That was significant because, after all those years in Boston, I still didn't know everybody from the Red Sox front office. So, it was good to see another organization and how they were run.

The Orioles, after decades of playing winning baseball, had fallen on hard times. Frank Robinson was their manager and was hoping I would provide veteran leadership to his young ball club. He also called the Orioles acquiring me a step in the right direction. Their general manager, Roland Hemond, took it a step further, telling reporters, "To have someone of Dwight's stature join our club is a big plus. He's such a fine all-around player and a future Hall of Famer."

And speaking of the reporters in Baltimore, they seemed more positive than what I was used to. In fact, one of them mentioned to me that I had led all of Major League Baseball in extra-base hits during the decade of the '80s. Somewhat astonished by this revelation, I told him, "I never knew that." To this day, I don't know why a reporter in Boston didn't share that with me. I had to find out in Baltimore. It was such a significant achievement. After all, there were some incredible hitters that played that entire '80s decade like Hall of Famers George Brett, Paul Molitor, Mike Schmidt, Robin Yount, Rickey Henderson, Jim Rice, Alan Trammell, Gary Carter, and Dave Winfield. So when I heard it from that Baltimore writer that I had more extra-base hits than any of them, it made me feel pretty good.

While I adjusted to my new place of business in Baltimore, Susan and the kids stayed in Lynnfield until the school year ended. But once June rolled around, we rented a beautiful condo in the historic Baltimore waterfront neighborhood of Canton—right across from Fort McHenry. With friends and parks and great restaurants nearby, we really enjoyed living there.

Meanwhile, the Orioles organization, aware of the boys' health issues, was very supportive. Justin, who was now 14 and had endured at least 20 surgeries by that time, continued to have benign tumors form under his skin. But the Orioles encouraged him to help the staff at Memorial Stadium on giveaway days—a continuation of the enjoyment he had in dealing with people from his time working at the Twins Souvenir store.

Despite the uphill challenges the Orioles had in '91, I got to play with some truly cerebral ballplayers and nice people. Our catcher, Bob Melvin, would go on to have a successful 20-year managerial career and is currently piloting the San Francisco Giants. And, of course, you had baseball royalty with the Ripken family—Cal Sr., Cal Jr., and Billy.

Cal Sr., one of the coaches, could look like Rambo with that stern look of his, but he was a sweet man and a great source of baseball knowledge. He once came up to me before a game when I was going through a slump and said, "You think you're finished, don't you?" At age 39, the thought had crossed my mind. But he very reassuringly told me, "You're *not* finished. You're just doing a few things wrong." A hard worker, he got me right in the cage and threw to me for 30 solid minutes. As it turned out, he was right—I was just doing some things that needed to be straightened out and was fine after that. His unyielding support helped get me back on track.

Billy, our second baseman, was one of the most hard-nosed players I ever played with. I always said Billy would dive on cement to catch a ball.

And then there was Cal Jr., a Hall of Famer and 19-time All-Star, who was one of the few bright spots on the '91 Orioles—winning AL MVP, All-Star Game MVP, and the All-Star Game Home Run Hitting Contest, as well as a Gold Glove Award at shortstop. He was also well on his way to a major league record for most consecutive games. So it was a great experience to be teammates with an all-time great like him.

But for me personally, nothing could rival my emotional return to Fenway Park on May 30 to start a four-game series against the Red Sox. Here I was, playing right field in an *Orioles* uniform—which felt really awkward—before sellout crowds in each of the games. The Fenway crowd was so generous with me. Almost every time I took the field and *every time* I came up to hit, they gave me standing ovations. I was deeply touched and would raise my hat or helmet to the crowd in gratitude all weekend long. There were even some fans wearing my replica Boston jersey, holding up signs that were derogatory toward the Red Sox who got kicked out of the ballpark. I always loved and had such a great rapport with Red Sox fans. Was I the best player they ever saw? No. But I played hard and gave everything I had. They appreciated me and I appreciated them right back. Their loyalty always meant so much to me.

But the one thing I was asked repeatedly from people on that trip that truly bothered me was, "Why did you leave Boston to go to Baltimore?" Their unawareness really surprised me. I had to tell them, "Well, I was fired, and I didn't have a job." Some of them were hard-pressed to believe I was released by the Red Sox. So, I would say, "Why would you think I would opt to go into free agency and go to Baltimore? I wanted to stay in Fenway." Having to explain this again and again bugged me to no end. It also reminded me how much I had wanted to finish my career in Boston. It was a tough time for me.

Thankfully, there was some solace in that I played well in front of my old teammates and fans in that series, and we took three out of the four games. And I would save my best for the final game of the series against Clemens. Facing a pitcher as great as Rocket was a challenge—no question about it. But in my first at-bat against him in the top of the second, with Joe Orsulak on first, I hit a line drive up the right field line. As the ball caromed off the fence in the corner, I raced around all the bases for what I thought was a two-run inside-the-park-home run, though it was later ruled a triple and an error on Brunansky. I don't know why it was scored like that because there didn't appear to be any missed plays. Nevertheless, it gave us a 2–0 lead.

In the top of the fourth, I would double to right field off Clemens. After the inning ended, as I ran by the mound, Roger sarcastically said to me, "What is it, Dewey, your birthday? What are you trying to do to me?!" Of course, it was all said in fun. I played with Roger for seven seasons, and we thoroughly enjoyed being teammates.

In my last at-bat against Rocket in the seventh, I hit a deep drive to right center field, but it was caught just in front of the fence. I couldn't help but think how sweet it would have been to add a home run to my day, but it wasn't to be.

And in my final plate appearance in the ninth, I popped out to third off Reardon. But the Fenway fans, knowing that was likely my last time at bat in the series, again rose to their feet and gave me a great sendoff. The gesture meant so much to me.

After that series ended, I was totally drained. It may have been a triumphant return to Fenway, but it was easily the most emotional four days I ever had on the playing field. I missed the fans, and there were still guys on the Red Sox who were my friends and a big part of my life. Despite the success the Orioles and I had on the field that series, the experience was difficult for me, and I was relieved when it was over.

Taking three out of four games in Boston was probably the highlight of an otherwise difficult season for the Orioles, as we would lose 95 games and finish in sixth place. The fall guy was Frank Robinson, replaced by Johnny Oates after a slow start in the first half of the campaign. While it was a privilege to play for a baseball legend and trailblazer like Robinson, I enjoyed playing for Johnny because of how well he used me and communicated with me. For instance, he'd tell me before the start of a four-game series, "You're going to be off the third game. But if a situation comes up late in the game with a certain pitcher out there, you're going to pinch-hit." That gave me plenty of heads-up to be ready just in case I was needed. And when called upon, I did a good job pinch-hitting. But first, I had to learn how to get ready and get into the mindset of being a pinch-hitter. So, I would go up in the clubhouse, loosen up, and then take these little tape balls and have a clubhouse guy flip them to me to swing at. We didn't have cages underneath the stands like teams have today, so this was the best way to get some cuts in.

After the '91 season ended, I worked hard to strengthen my back and was as healthy as I had been in at least three or four years. My back, thankfully, was now a non-issue. And even though I would start spring training as a 40-year-old, I had it in my mind to play at least one or two more seasons. Meanwhile, the Orioles were talking with me about as many as three more years. Hemond, one of the classiest guys in all of baseball, pressed me in the off-season, telling me, "We need to know. We want to make a decision here regarding an extension." I told him what I was thinking and said, "I'll let you know soon enough. But let's plan on one year and address an extension halfway through the season after we see how everything goes." I didn't know for sure if I wanted to play more than one year at that point. I thought by spring training I might have a better idea and could share my thoughts then. As it turned out, that was probably a mistake.

In the early days of spring training in 1992, the Orioles worked out at Twin Lakes Park in Sarasota, which was an older facility that didn't drain well, leaving the ground soft after it rained. I ended up pulling a calf muscle, which I had never done before, because the field was so spongy. As it was healing, I said something to Oates that I regret saying to this day. There was a stipulation in my contract that if they decided to cut me during spring training, they had to do it early so I could catch on with another team. I don't know why that was put into my contract, but it was probably originally thought to be in my best interest. So, a few days after the injury, while Oates had one of his meetings with me to discuss how he was going to use me that season, I really put my foot in my mouth. Being way too honest with him, I said, "Johnny, I just want to let you know about something that's in my contract." Oates cut me off and said, "I don't want to know anything." But Oates was a really neat guy and I trusted him, so I opened my big mouth and told him what was in the clause.

Sure enough, the next day Johnny came over to me and said, "You've got to get it going with that calf. I've got to see what you can do."

With the calf still an issue, I stayed out of the field and DH'd a couple of days later in a game against the Cardinals at Al Lang Stadium in St. Petersburg. In my second and last at-bat of the game, with a runner on second and two outs, I hit a bullet through the middle for an RBI single. I had my timing down and was feeling really good at the plate. And most importantly, I showed Johnny I could play.

So, the next morning, I was completely shell-shocked when Hemond called me in and said, "We're going to release you." Being a Christian, I didn't have any animosity toward either Oates or Hemond over it. I blamed myself more than anything else. I didn't have to give them the information about my clause. I just felt I could trust Johnny and talk about anything with him.

In fairness, I really don't know all the details of what went on behind the scenes in releasing me. Were they concerned I was damaged goods? Did they want to go with a younger right fielder? Was it to save money? I never found out for sure. But now I had a problem. Other teams were afraid to even entertain signing me because I was released so early in spring training. Their natural thinking was that something serious must have been wrong with me for that to have happened.

So, just like that, my 20-year major league career was over. It was one filled with great achievements, accomplishments, and memories. But when looking back at the challenges on the field and in my personal life—the beanballs to the head and all those sleepless nights in hospitals worrying about and comforting my sons—I overcame an awful lot to have the successful career that I did. In my mind, it was a career defined by perseverance and always having the presence of God and Christ in me. I cannot illustrate this anymore than what was written in the wonderful poem, "Footprints in the Sand."

> One night I dreamed a dream.
> As I was walking along the beach with my Lord.
> Across the dark sky flashed scenes from my life.
> For each scene, I noticed two sets of footprints in the sand,
> One belonging to me and one to my Lord.
>
> After the last scene of my life flashed before me,
> I looked back at the footprints in the sand.
> I noticed that at many times along the path of my life,
> especially at the very lowest and saddest times,
> there was only one set of footprints.
>
> This really troubled me, so I asked the Lord about it.
> "Lord, you said once I decided to follow you,
> You'd walk with me all the way.
> But I noticed that during the saddest and most
>   troublesome times of my life,
> there was only one set of footprints.
> I don't understand why, when I needed You the most,
>   You would leave me."

He whispered, "My precious child, I love you and will
    never leave you
Never, ever, during your trials and testings.
When you saw only one set of footprints,
It was then that I carried you."

I may have endured some very difficult days, but it was during those times when walking with God—and there were only two footprints in the sand instead of four—it was then that He carried me. Without God's comfort, I would have never succeeded the way I did.

And now, after all those years of playing ball, it was time to go home.

CHAPTER 22

GIVING BACK TO THE GAME

"DEWEY, WE'VE BOTH HAD GREAT CAREERS," former All-Star third baseman Buddy Bell told me in 1992 at the Birmingham Barons' Hoover Metropolitan Stadium. "You played 20 years, and I played 18. But that's all over. Now it's time to bring all that knowledge and all those skills we have and teach these kids the right way to play baseball."

It was at that very moment that I knew what my post-baseball-playing career mission was—to pass on what I had learned and give back to the game.

Buddy was running the Chicago White Sox minor league system and was my boss after I accepted a job as a roving outfield and batting instructor with their organization. Bell was great to work for and had an excellent eye for talent. As we continued to talk, he said, "See that guy at third base? He's going to the big leagues." I looked over and went, "*That* third baseman?" I mentioned the kid's name and Buddy goes, "No, the *coach* at third. He's going to be a big-league manager." That coach's name was Terry Francona. Terry would go on to become a great manager and would lead the Red Sox to two world championships and Cleveland to a pennant.

Prior to accepting the job with the White Sox, my agent, Jack Sands, and I met with Red Sox general manager Lou Gorman and team president John Harrington. The Red Sox had promised me a position within the organization upon my retirement and we were interested to see what they had in mind for me. They offered me the manager's job with the Class A-Advanced Salem (Virginia) Red Sox of the Carolina League. While it was a great offer if I ever wanted to get on a big-league managerial track, I didn't want that. I had just played 24 years in professional baseball and largely missed seeing my family grow up. A job with Salem would have meant eight months of going to spring training and managing a full season—plus riding the buses again—without seeing much of Susan or the kids. I wasn't ready for that. Instead, I asked if a roving instructor's job was available. Lou said nothing like that would be opening up for the foreseeable future.

So, Jack had a Plan B. He was really close with Jerry Reins-dorf, the longtime owner of both the White Sox and the Chicago Bulls, and he set up a meeting with him. Reinsdorf, a very kind individual, asked me, "What do you want to do?" I said, "I'd like to just rove." He asked, "Well, how many days a month do you want to work?" I said, "Ten to twelve. That's all I have time for right now. I can work with your outfielders on defense, and I can work with everyone on their hitting." Jerry leaned back in his chair and said, "Okay, but on your trips home, I want you to connect through Chicago O'Hare, leave two hours between flights, and I'll meet you there. We'll have a cup of coffee and then you can continue home." That was easy, as I would be flying back mostly from their Double-A team in Birmingham and Triple-A team in Nashville, and occasionally from Sarasota, the home base of the Florida State League.

And sure enough, that's what Jerry and I did. Here was a guy worth hundreds of millions of dollars, the owner of the Michael Jordan–Scottie Pippen dynastic Bulls as well as a White Sox team that featured Frank Thomas, winner of back-to-back MVPs during that period, wanting to know how the little guy that he just signed to a minor league contract was doing. Usually wearing a short-sleeve white shirt with an unlit cigar in his mouth, he'd jot down notes on index cards, and then we would meet again two or three weeks later. To me, it showed a lot about him and his character. He was very involved and was one of the nicest people I ever met in baseball. I truly enjoyed my time with him. And I loved the roving job itself, working with some promising up-and-coming players like a young Mike Cameron, who would go on to have a long, solid big-league career.

After the '93 season ended, Bell accepted an offer to be the bench coach for the Indians. With Buddy gone from the White Sox organization, Reinsdorf wanted me to take over Bell's job and run the minor leagues. It was intriguing because I was really starting to become familiar with the players and the system. Plus, I was confident I could do a good job and would certainly be very well compensated.

But around the same time, I got a call from Donnie Baylor, manager of the Colorado Rockies, who wanted me to be his hitting coach. I was really confused and conflicted about what I should do, so I called Bell for his input. Buddy said, "Dewey, anytime you have a chance to go to the major leagues, you *go* to the major leagues."

So, I declined the job with the White Sox and joined Donnie with the Rockies, taking a pay cut to go to the big leagues.

The Rockies were an expansion team in just their second year of existence in 1994, but they already had a strong lineup. My former Red Sox teammate Ellis Burks was there along with the "Big Cat," Andrés Galarraga, a huge man and a great talent. They also had other power hitters like Dante Bichette, Vinny Castilla, and Howard Johnson. Being their hitting coach was a terrific experience.

But, in hindsight, I probably should have taken the White Sox minor league director's position. There was a major league strike in 1994 that began on August 12 that would cancel the rest of the season—including the World Series. Plus, all the time away from my family was taking its toll and I needed to be home.

So, I made the decision to resign from my post, take a step back, and reevaluate my situation. But I felt very good about the work I did with the Rockies and was thrilled they went to the postseason in 1995. And I was happy for Baylor, who won the Manager of the Year Award.

—————————

Back at home, we were at an inflection point with the kids, and I felt the time was right to take a self-imposed hiatus from the game for what would turn out to be the next six years. Kirstin had graduated from Lynnfield High School and would begin a new phase of her life as a student at Endicott College. Justin would soon also graduate from high school, attend Curry College, earn a bachelor's degree in communications, and begin work for the Massachusetts Department of Transportation before settling in as a host at the Capital Grille restaurant in Burlington for many years—a job he loved.

But most importantly at the time, Timothy was suffering agonizing pain and limited sight in his left eye—a side-effect from NF—and needed all our support. He had been taking Percocet for years to alleviate some of the eye pain and, of course, we were always concerned he would become addicted to the drug. But now the pain had become unbearable, and we needed to act. We took him to see a world-renowned specialist who examined his eye and ran a series of tests. He described Timothy's condition as like having a nail in your eye that you can't pull out. He then put drops in his eye to numb it. A moment passed before Timothy turned to the specialist and us with a sense of relief and said, "I don't have any more pain." But the prognosis was not good, and the doctor delivered some devastating news. "Timothy has a sick eye, and it needs to come out."

We had no choice. Timothy couldn't continue with the level of pain he was enduring, so we moved forward with the procedure. The specialized surgery, which would take place in Philadelphia, was unique in that no other specialist was performing it. It entailed taking a little muscle off the top of the rear end, rolling it up, and then attaching it to the muscles in the eye, so it would be like a ball. So, if the muscles in your eye moved, the ball would move, too. A lens was made for Timothy, but since it didn't have much movement, the procedure didn't have the full effect it was supposed to have. Still, Timothy was able to keep his sense of humor. After a couple of days in the hospital, we were on the plane heading home when he turned to me—still in pain from where they removed the muscle from his rear end—and said, "Dad, you're not going to call me "Ass Eye" from now on, are you?"

We both had a good laugh. But that's the kind of sense of humor Timothy had, even in the toughest of times. And it certainly served him well.

By the year 2000, NF had been a part of our lives for a quarter of a century. That year, Susan and I decided we wanted to bring about a greater awareness of the disease to the public, so we became involved in supporting a Burlington, Massachusetts–based organization called Neurofibromatosis Northeast, which is affiliated with the national NF Network. The organization works to find treatments and a cure for NF, as well as creating programs and resources to help patients and families cope with the challenges that come with the disease. It was always surprising to us that NF afflicts three times as many people as those with muscular dystrophy and cystic fibrosis *combined*, but few people not impacted by it have ever heard of the disease. We wanted to do our part to see if we could change that.

We began working with a wonderful person named Karen Peluso, the executive director of Neurofibromatosis Northeast, who has been raising funds and working diligently as an advocate for NF research since 1982. NF Northeast, mostly through special fundraising events like golf tournaments, has provided more than $3 million in research grants since its inception. Karen became involved in NF Northeast after her daughter Mia underwent surgery to remove a large tumor in her abdomen caused by NF. Karen, like us, was stunned by how devastating the manifestations of NF could be—progressing from learning disabilities to hearing loss to blindness to cancer to death—as well as the lack of information and scientific research being done on it.

That was where I felt that I, as a former Red Sox player with children afflicted by NF, could make an impact by volunteering my time at various events to help raise money. And I was also able to reach out to The Yawkey Foundation, which is committed to continuing the legacy of former Red Sox owners Tom and Jean Yawkey through its financial support of worthy causes. As a result, The Yawkey Foundation agreed to give NF Northeast a sizable grant every other year. However, the grant was given to us under the stipulation that none of it would go into NF research. Instead, every penny needed to be used to get the word out and educate people about the disease. The conditions given to us by The Yawkey Foundation on how to use their grant made perfect sense to us.

When healthy enough, Justin would help us in our efforts. In fact, even when we couldn't attend an NF Northeast event, Justin would go on his own and give assistance where needed. So, as a family, we were doing our part in the battle against NF.

I would rejoin the Red Sox organization in 2001. The kids were young adults now and it seemed like the right time to get back in the game. After meeting with Red Sox general manager Dan Duquette and manager Joe Kerrigan, they wanted me to work in the minor leagues as a roving hitting coordinator. I told them, "I'll do that. I *want* to do that. But I only want to do Double-A and Triple-A. I can't handle more than that with all the players. But I can bring in someone else to handle the other levels."

They agreed and I brought in Victor Rodriguez, a very talented guy who I could trust to cover hitting with the lower levels of our minor league system. He would end up a part of the Red Sox organization in various roles for a total of 17 years before moving on and becoming the Cleveland assistant hitting coach following the 2017 season.

As it turned out, I wouldn't stay a roving hitting coordinator for long. About three weeks later that October, Duquette called me and said, "We want you to be our major league hitting coach for the 2002 season." At first, I was apprehensive about the time commitment and took a couple of weeks to mull it over with my family. But after talking it through with Susan and after the Red Sox really made it worthwhile—probably offering me the highest salary of any hitting coach in baseball—I accepted and was looking forward to this new challenge.

But a major shakeup took place the very first week of spring training when, on February 27, 2002, a new ownership group led by John Henry and Tom Werner completed their record $660 million purchase of the Red Sox. The landmark deal ended seven decades of ownership by the Yawkey family and its trust. What it also did was lead to the quick dismissal of Duquette, who was fired from his general manager's post within 24 hours of the sale and was replaced by Mike Port. Five days after Duquette was let go, Kerrigan was also fired, and Grady Little was brought in as the new manager. So, the two guys who were responsible for hiring me as the Red Sox hitting coach just months before were now gone.

But the shakeup wasn't over yet. Grady wanted some of his own coaches, which was totally understandable. So, he reassigned our pitching coach Ralph Treuel near the end of spring training, replacing him with Tony Cloninger. The rest of the coaches, including myself, were safe—at least for a time. In fact, there was a rumor that Grady might replace me with one of his friends in the game, our bench coach Mike Stanley. But Little met with me in his office and asked, "Do you want to be my hitting coach?" I told him I did. He reassured me, saying, "I don't know how these rumors got started about you. They weren't true."

So, after all the chaos that surrounded Red Sox spring training, things eventually settled down and everyone was able concentrate on their respective roles on the ball club. I really enjoyed being back in uniform with the Red Sox. It was like coming home again.

What I loved most about being the Red Sox hitting coach was working with the players. Up and down the lineup, we had guys with great work ethics. One of my favorites was Johnny Damon, whom we had just acquired as a free agent. Damon was the ultimate gamer and one of the toughest players I've ever been around. One time, when our first base coach Tommy Harper was on bereavement leave, I filled in for him. Damon got on and had to dive back into first base. When he got up, one of his fingers was pointing sideways—completely dislocated. He was holding it up and I went, "Oh, God." So, Grady came out and said to Damon, "Come on, Johnny, let's go." And Damon said, "No, I can run. I can score. I'm fine." But I said, "Johnny, come on, you've got to come out." So, he reluctantly walked off the field, pulled his finger, and put it back in the joint. He didn't play the next day, but he played every game after that.

I worked hard with Damon, who had an off year at the plate in 2001 with Oakland following a terrific season with the Kansas City Royals the year before. I noticed Johnny was raising his hands too soon and letting go of the bat at contact with his top hand, so I got him to hold on to the bat with both hands and finishing high. He responded really well and had an All-Star season in 2002, increasing his batting average by 30 points and leading the league in triples. And, of course, Damon would become a folk hero in Boston just two years later by playing a key role in the Red Sox winning the World Series.

I also took an immediate liking to Shea Hillenbrand, just a second-year third baseman at the time, who was a quick learner. Shea was a big, strong kid who I worked hard with on pitch selection and working counts. Once he started working the counts to his advantage, staying within himself and patiently waiting for his pitch to hit, he quickly blossomed into a good hitter, making the All-Star team that year.

And I was most impressed with the great attitude, work ethic, and toughness of Jason Varitek, our young catcher who was already showing signs of being a great team leader and a favorite amongst the pitchers and coaches for his preparation and knowledge of the game. "Tek" would go on to become a big part of two world-championship Red Sox teams and currently has a role on the coaching staff.

I was able to offer my knowledge and experience to everyone on the club—no matter their level of experience or skill—without being overbearing. And that included veterans like Rickey Henderson and Nomar Garciaparra. With Rickey, who was 43 years old but still had a quick bat, I could offer him encouragement if he got into a slump and dissuade him from thinking his career might be over because of it. I could do that with him because I had those same thoughts during my last big-league season with the Orioles. With Nomar, I didn't need to go too deep. I never saw a guy hit the ball on the perfect part of the bat so consistently. He probably used only three inches of the barrel, which is pretty special.

I was also able to help the guys better understand how to deal with and embrace being an athlete in Boston. My best advice, whether they were an average or above-average player, was to always bust their rear end and they would quickly earn the respect of our demanding, passionate fans.

Despite the positive strides some of the guys made with their hitting and the club winning 93 games—an 11-game improvement over the previous campaign—more moves were made to the coaching staff after the season. This time around, Harper, our bullpen coach Bob Kipper, and I were all fired, with Stanley deciding to resign for family reasons. Grady brought the coaches he was dismissing into his office and gave us the news with very little further communication about his decision. It was obvious he just wanted his own people on his staff which, again, I understood. In my case, it probably didn't help that Nomar hit "only" .310— even if it was an improvement over his previous injury-riddled season. But this was a guy that hit .357 and .372 back in 1999 and 2000, respectively, so I suppose I was made the fall guy because he didn't approach those numbers again in 2002.

In hindsight, that was a tough season. But I was glad I got to know the great group of guys we had on that club.

Fortunately, however, right after I was fired, I was re-hired by the Red Sox to work in player development. It didn't hurt that I had a great relationship with the club's new president, Larry Lucchino, going back to my one season in Baltimore where he was also president. I was thrilled to remain in the Red Sox organization. One of the requirements of my new position was to work in uniform with our younger players during spring training in Fort

Myers. Spring training was great because I was rubbing shoulders with the minor league guys on the Red Sox 40-man roster, so when I showed up at our Triple-A Pawtucket facility during the season, they already knew me. Plus, I stayed in regular touch with them throughout their season, as I was able to watch and talk with them about all their minor league games, which were Skyped to me via computer.

In the meantime, our big-league club was at the dawn of a great 15-year run. In 2003, the Red Sox would take the Yankees to the 11th inning of the seventh game of the ALCS before its season ended on an Aaron Boone home run.

At last, in 2004, all the pain that the Red Sox and their fans endured over the previous 86 years would end when Boston won the World Series for the first time since 1918. I felt the excitement and the joy of the championship because the new owners made all of us feel that we were part of it. And they showed their appreciation the following season in the greatest way. I was making an appearance up in the Legends' Suite at Fenway Park when, suddenly, a camera crew came in and I was presented with a beautiful wooden box from the owners. When I opened it, there was a 2004 World Series ring with the inscriptions 2004 GREATEST COMEBACK IN HISTORY on one side and EVANS P.D. (Player Development) on the other side. It was a total surprise. And what made that moment even sweeter was having Timothy with me, who was equally blown away by it.

Everybody in the Red Sox organization would get a ring. These owners are so good. They don't miss any opportunity to show how much they care and are so much fun to be around.

I'm shocked when some people ask me things like, "How did you feel about the Sox winning the World Series in 2004?" or "Are you jealous that they won?" I always say, "What do you mean? It was awesome!" I played for some power-packed Red Sox teams in the mid-'70s and late '80s that should have been good enough to win two or three world championships. My only regret in my baseball career was not being able to bring a World Series title to the Red Sox and their fans. We had our opportunities, but we couldn't get the job done. But these guys did and that's the bottom line. And the way they did it—down three games to none against the Yankees and coming back to win four straight, then sweeping the St. Louis Cardinals in the World Series—was remarkable. I was so proud to be part of the organization when the Red Sox finally won it all.

The Red Sox would win it all again in 2007, but what made that championship even sweeter wouldn't occur until Opening Day 2008 at Fenway Park. The Red Sox flew me up from Florida so I could catch Bill Buckner's ceremonial first pitch. Buck had skipped the 2005 Opening Day celebration of the 2004 championship to avoid all the attention he thought he would draw because of his infamous error in the '86 World Series. And he didn't return to Fenway for the twentieth anniversary celebration of our '86 pennant in which he received the loudest ovation of any of us in absentia. Buck still felt deep scars from all the backlash he endured from our '86 World Series loss. But thanks to some prodding from our public relations director Dick Bresciani, Buck decided the time was finally right following two Red Sox world championships to return to Boston.

Overcome with emotion and with tears welling up in his eyes, Buck walked slowly onto the field toward the mound as the fans rose in unison and gave him a long, thunderous ovation. I met him halfway, embraced him, and told him how touched I was to catch his first pitch. Now he's crying like a little kid. The fans' reaction to having him back meant the world to him. The true fans knew our losing the '86 World Series wasn't his fault. They knew his heart and what a gamer he was. It was finally time for

Red Sox fans to look back at all Buck did for the team and say, "Thank you!"

Buck was one of my dearest friends in baseball and I miss him dearly since he passed away from Lewy body dementia in 2019. I spoke to him just a few months before he died and was shocked by how fast-moving Lewy body dementia is. Buck will always be a Red Sox legend. But more importantly to me, he will always be a great friend.

After all these years, I'm still in Red Sox player development and couldn't be happier doing what I'm doing for them. At my age, clubs usually try to phase you out. Not here. They ask more and more of me, and it makes me feel proud. I've made an impact on hundreds of prospects over the years and my greatest reward is seeing them succeed and do well in "the Show."

I have thoroughly enjoyed working with and developing too many young players to mention here, but one that really stands out was outfielder Jackie Bradley Jr. The Red Sox drafted him in the first round of the 2011 amateur draft and then signed him later that year. Jackie was one of the stars of the South Carolina Gamecocks baseball team that won National Championships in 2010 and 2011. The first time I met him, he said, "Hi, I'm Jackie Bradley Jr." I said, "Yeah, I know who you are, Jackie." And he said, "I heard you had a pretty good arm." I went, "Well, I worked hard. I did have a pretty good arm." And he said, "I want you to know that I've got a pretty good arm, too." I'll never forget that initial exchange with this 21-year-old kid who would develop into a fine major leaguer for us. I admired the confidence he showed in his very humble way. He just knew he had a pretty good arm and wanted to make sure I knew it, too. I loved that. Jackie was a great kid—one of the special ones.

Being part of the Red Sox has also afforded me unique opportunities away from the game. In 2011, I made my Hollywood debut in the Farrelly brothers' movie *Hall Pass* as the Maggie character's (played by Jenna Fischer) father. But I must confess, it was probably the hardest day of work I ever had. Peter and Bobby Farrelly had originally reached out to me through the Red Sox about playing a part in the movie. Not knowing what the movie was about, I said to them, "Can I see the lines?"

So after reading the lines, we spoke again and I told them, "Yeah, I can do that." However, I assumed I was going to have a teleprompter to help me out, making it a no-brainer. All they told me was, "Just learn your lines"—there was nothing about having them memorized. This was on a Monday, and I had to be in Atlanta for filming that Thursday, so it wasn't like I had a lot of time to learn them by heart. When I arrived on a set made to look like Cape Cod that Thursday morning, I didn't see any teleprompters around. I knew right away how difficult it was going to be for me to walk, talk, try to act normal, remember everyone's lines, and know when to chime in.

We ended up working until seven o'clock that night. There were several instances when we executed our roles perfectly, but because some jet was flying over or a siren went off or a car honked, they would go, "Cut! Got to do it over again." And it was never just one line we had to re-do, but the entire segment. One of the stars, Christina Applegate, who is even prettier in person than she is on-screen, was a great help to me. When it got to be five o'clock and I was so worn out I became tongue-tied, she took me aside and gave me some great pointers. After that, I nailed it.

They had wanted me to curse in the film, but I told them that I didn't swear. So, it was kind of funny when, every time I saw

Peter or Bobby in the ensuing years, they'd always ask me, "You're still not swearing, right?" It kind of became our inside joke.

––––––––––––

The Red Sox would win the World Series again in 2013 and 2018 to give them four world championships this century—more than any other team in baseball. And just like in 2004 and 2007, *everyone* in the organization received a World Series ring. The current ownership group proves again and again how they take care of their own. I've seen many occasions where former players were only here four or five years and how the team still takes care of them in so many ways. To be called a Boston Red Sox comes with great respect, honor, and loyalty.

The year 2024 marks my 43rd year in the Red Sox organization and, perhaps more than anyone, I can relate to how powerful the history of the club truly is. I have tremendous appreciation for its traditions and embrace the emotions that come with playing in Boston over a lengthy period of time. I may have been raised in Hawaii and grew up in Southern California, but I became a New Englander. Susan and I chose to stay in the Boston area to raise our family instead of moving back West where we both came from. I cannot begin to describe how much I loved the Dodgers as a kid. I saw them play at the Los Angeles Memorial Coliseum after they moved from Brooklyn. I saw them at Dodger Stadium in Chavez Ravine. There were so many great memories growing up watching that team. But for as much as I loved the Dodgers as a kid, that's how much I love the Red Sox as *an older kid* now.

I'll be a Boston Red Sox until I pass on. I would like to think that. Afterall, even at my current age, I'm still in uniform, can still communicate with the players, and still have my balance. But most importantly, I still have my love for this great game.

CHAPTER 23

PEACE AND EMPTINESS

Life isn't supposed to work this way. Seeing your grandparents, then your parents, and perhaps even your spouse pass on before you is the natural order of things. A parent should never have to endure the heartache of burying their own child. But within a one-year period, Susan and I would lose both Justin and Timothy—an almost incomprehensible emotional trauma.

With our sons' relentless battle against NF, and with the more than 40 surgeries each of them would have over the course of their lives, we always knew the time might come when we would have to say goodbye to them. But we were too busy trying to keep them alive to think much about that.

In 2018, Justin developed a glioblastoma brain tumor that we didn't want to do a biopsy on. That was because the tumor was located at the base of his brain, and the surgeons couldn't get rid of it without damaging the brain. Shortly thereafter, he suffered a stroke that could have been caused by the tumor. After the stroke, he was gone within a year at just 42 years old.

A devout Christian with an open, kind heart for everyone, Justin passed away in hospice care, ironically on Easter Sunday in 2019. He had taught Sunday school at Calvary Christian Church in Lynnfield for years, and one of his great joys was spending time with children and telling them stories about Jesus. And right up until the end of his life, he kept his sense of humor. He would call us from his home in Stoneham, and Susan would answer the phone and kiddingly say abruptly, "What do you want?!" He just laughed and laughed. Then I would get on the phone, and he'd go, "Hey *old man*, how you doing?" By keeping things as lighthearted as we could, we stayed strong for each other throughout this most difficult period of our lives.

Justin had always gotten along well with everyone. And he never said anything bad about anybody. Ten days after he passed, I went to get my car washed. As I paid the guy at the drive-through, he gave me a double-look and goes, "You're *Justin's dad*, aren't you?" Not Dwight Evans, but Justin's dad. I said, "Yeah." And the man said, "I really liked Justin. He was such a great and funny guy. I just wanted to tell you that." And you know what—that was a cookie I really needed at that time.

However, we would go through the same level of sorrow 10 months later when Timothy passed away at 47 in Fort Myers. At least with Timothy, I was so glad that he had found happiness and fulfillment in his life six years before when he'd married a lovely woman named Susana from Jakarta. They met through a Christian online site and, after about a year, Timothy flew from Boston to London to Singapore to Jakarta—a 33-hour trip—to meet her. After two weeks with her, he flew home from Jakarta via Tokyo and San Francisco, and then back to Boston—completing his trip around the world—and said to Susan and me, "She's the one I want to marry." It was a good time in our lives to see him get married and then to watch them get to know and learn more about one another. And when he later got sick, she was there for him. It surely wasn't her dream to come all the way to this country and have her husband's health deteriorate, but she stayed by his side and was of great comfort to him until the end.

Unlike Justin, who could no longer combat the effects of NF, it was Timothy's decision to stop the treatments that were keeping him alive. He was living with a great deal of pain and, because his balance was off, had to walk with a cane—but he was still able to manage. But then one day we were at his doctor's office and, after the physician told us how pleased he was with how his glioblastoma brain cancer was under control, Timothy stood up, looked right at him, and said, "I'm done." Susan and I looked at him in bewilderment. "What do you mean you're *done*?" I asked him. And Timothy said, "I don't want any more treatment. I'm tired of living like this." For as difficult as it was for Susan and me to hear that, we supported his decision. Still, it was a sobering moment. Death is hard. For as much as we wanted to be supportive of his choice, it didn't come easily for us. We had just lost our youngest son and now we were going to lose our only other son.

But then something occurred just 10 days before Timothy passed away that gave us all some comfort. He was receiving hospice care in his home, and Susan and I would visit him for as long as we could each day. On this one visit, as we were leaving, I kissed Timothy on the forehead and he said, "Dad, I had a dream last night." I said, "What about, Tim?" And he goes, "I had a dream that I was looking up at Jesus and he put His hand out and, while He was pulling me up, I saw Justin behind Him." Timothy was in a weakened state, and it had taken at least half a minute for him to get those few words out. I said, "Well, what happened after that, Tim?" And he said softly, "I woke up." After that dream, Timothy wasn't afraid anymore of passing from this life to another life. He knew where he was going. And he knew there would be no more pain. Still, Susan and I continued to pray that God would heal him—just as we had done for Justin—right up until he took his last breath. But that wasn't in God's plans.

While I am at peace knowing that both Justin and Timothy are now in heaven, watching our two sons die in our presence was a heavy thing to handle. But those are also moments—for as heartbreaking as they were—in which I was glad I was there. I couldn't imagine if their lives were taken in another way where I wouldn't have the chance to say goodbye.

But still, on particularly difficult days when the reality of them being gone hits me especially hard, I miss them so much that I break down. It's during those times when I have to force myself to recall when they were both very sick and how I didn't want them suffering anymore. This way of thinking provides some relief. But then there's this emptiness that sometimes takes over, which is hard to explain. There's still that hurt that we don't have them anymore. They were not only our sons, but they were also our friends. And I feel badly that they both never experienced what it's like to have children and a normal life. But on the other side of it, I'm also thankful we had them in our lives for as long as we did. And I think that's hard for most people that have never lost a child to understand.

Another thing I found is how difficult it is for some people to express themselves properly at funerals—as was the case at our sons' services. They say things like, "Oh, they're in a better place." Well, we already know that. I don't need to be reminded of that. Or worse, they'll say, "We know what you're going through." Well, how could they possibly know? One time, after getting tired of repeatedly hearing that, I responded to someone with, "Oh, you lost a child?" And the person said somewhat sheepishly, "Well, no, but we have a friend that did." If well-intentioned people don't know what to say, the advice I would give them would be to just put their hand on the grieving person's shoulder, look at them eye-to-eye, and say, "I've got nothing, but I care deeply about you and hurt for you. And I'm praying for you." That's all you need to do. That speaks volumes. Then leave it alone and move on. It's a lesson in etiquette at a funeral or around people that are going through a tough time.

With people I know who are aware that I'm a Christian, I've often been asked, "How did losing your sons affect your faith?" And I tell them, "Not at all. If anything, it makes it stronger because my boys know Christ personally." In fact, I would love to know what the boys are doing now and what paradise in heaven is like for them, because I totally believe in that. When I tell people that, they'll often say, "Well, then it'll be great when you can see them again." And Susan and I both look forward to that. We're not in any hurry to go, but when God wants us, we're ready.

As was the case with Justin, in the weeks and months that followed Timothy's passing, we received cards and letters from people with glowing things to say about Timothy and what he meant to their lives. One letter was from a grown man named Brian who grew up on our Lynnfield block but had long since moved away and now has a wife and four children of his own. The man wrote how when he was a youngster, a group of five neighborhood kids tried to gang up on him on the street and Timothy, a couple of years older than Brian, stood behind him and kept the other boys away. The letter went on to say, "I just wanted to tell you what Tim did for me. He stuck up for me, protected me, and he looked out for me." Susan and I never knew Timothy did that. It sounded like something he would do because so many kids put him down because he didn't look like everyone else. But he did that for this kid. It meant so much for Susan and me to hear that story and what Timothy meant to Brian growing up. It was a reminder to us of how great a person Timothy was and how much he cared about people.

From my baseball world, I can't say enough about how much I appreciated the concern that came from Bruce Hurst. When I lost both of my sons, he stayed in touch with me throughout and wanted to know how I was doing. Bruce would call during those toughest moments of my life—not easy calls to make. But he would do it, and that is something I will never forget.

I also heard from Yaz, my best friend in baseball, after Timothy's passing. If anyone could relate to what I was going through, it was Carl. He lost his own son, Michael, at age 44 to blood clots after hip surgery in 2004. His taking the time to make a very difficult phone call to me meant so much.

But Yaz would do even more. The day I reported to spring training in Fort Myers less than two weeks after Timothy's passing for my Red Sox player development job (yes, baseball was still, after all these years, therapeutic for me), I went to right field to shag fly balls with some of the players. And out of nowhere, completely unexpected, Yaz appears and starts walking toward me in the outfield. Surprised to see him, I said, "*Carl!*" But he didn't say a word. As Yaz got closer, I extended my right hand to shake his, but instead of shaking it, he put both of his arms around me to console me. Words didn't need to be said. His action spoke volumes. It was an act of friendship that gave me great comfort at a time when I needed it most.

Yaz and I hung out in the outfield for a while before walking off the field together—talking and relating to one another only as two fathers that lost children can.

It's special friends like Yaz who help me a lot.

CHAPTER 24

LIFE GOES ON

W ITH A HEAVY HEART but a strong faith to carry on with a life filled with blessings, I still look at each day as a gift. I've had a baseball career that most people could only dream about. I've been happily married to Susan—a beautiful woman who's been my "everything"—for more than 53 years. And I have a healthy daughter, Kirstin, who has blessed us with four wonderful grandchildren—Ryan, Michael, Alyssa, and Darren Berardino—of whom I am extremely proud. And my current role with the Red Sox keeps me energized and feeling young.

I also feel so fortunate to connect with diehard Red Sox fans at venues like the Legends Suite at Fenway Park. It allows me to talk baseball with groups who always impress me with their knowledge of the game and appreciation of Red Sox history. A subject that often gets raised by fans is why I'm not in the Baseball Hall of Fame. It's flattering to hear that. I truly believe that as I was coming up for voting by the Baseball Writers Association of America (BBWAA) in the late '90s, the thinking was that I was on the bubble offensively, but that my defensive ability as a complete player would put me over the top. But that was the beginning of the steroid era in baseball, when Sammy Sosa and Mark McGwire started hitting more than 60 home runs a season and the writers' offensive benchmarks for statistics like home runs were raised dramatically from the era in which I played. Suddenly, writers were saying that hitting 400 home runs was no longer the criteria for Hall of Fame consideration—now it was 500 or 550. As a result, I fell off the ballot quickly.

I've long believed a player should be evaluated for Hall of Fame consideration based on the era in which they played. So now there is a Contemporary Baseball Era Committee that meets every three years to consider candidates whose greatest contribution to the game were realized from 1980 to the present era. Well, even though I led the American League in home runs and all of Major League baseball in extra-base hits during the 1980s—and was right there in RBIs and runs scored—I wasn't even on the Contemporary Era Committee's ballot for 2023. I just didn't understand that logic and it kind of bothered me at the time. But I'm not going to lose any sleep over it. It is what it is. I'm proud of my performance during the era in which I played and if it happens that one day I get selected to the Hall of Fame, that would be a great honor. It would further justify all my hard work and dedication, and that what I did on the playing field meant something. But if it doesn't happen, I'll still be a Hall of Famer in heaven.

All that I've gone through in my personal life and continue to go through today gives me the proper perspective on things. In 2022, Susan was diagnosed with Somatostatinoma, an extremely rare, highly cancerous malignant tumor that was above her pancreas. It affects just 1 in 40 million people. It couldn't be treated with chemotherapy or radiation because it's so rare. Instead, surgeons just had to cut the tumor out during a highly difficult surgery in a sensitive area.

I worried that I might lose her. There was a point when I finally thought, *Well, I'm looking at life without Susan.* I honestly didn't know what I would do without her. It was a terrible time.

But then I came to realize that we had been married for more than 52 years and thought, *How long does it last? Fifty-two years is quite a run. And I am truly thankful for that.* That being said, I wanted to be with her until the end of time.

Mercifully, my prayers were answered, the surgery was a success, and she's doing much better now. Every day we spend together is a little more precious after what she went through. We try to spend more time together and don't take anything for granted. We take each day as it comes. But if something were to pop up again, I don't think she would want to go through that invasive surgery again. She knows where she's going after this life and wants to see her boys. She looks forward to that and I do, too.

I truly believe that a wife is a gift from God. I've been blessed to have Susan in my life ever since we met when we were both 15 years old. She watched me play high school ball, then came to the minor leagues with me, was by my side throughout my 20 seasons in the major leagues, and continued to be supportive when I decided to go into coaching and player development. I never would have lasted as long as I did in professional baseball without her. The baseball life can be hard on marriages—especially with all the travel—and I get asked occasionally how mine has survived the test of time. I always say that marriage is not 50/50. You both have to give 100 percent. Marriage is work and isn't easy. You do and say stupid things and argue and bicker over nonsense. But we stayed together and now, after all these years, we're so close that we finish one another's sentences and know what the other person is thinking. And for us, the bedrock of our union is our relationship with God. It's hard to explain, but it's like the wind—you can't see it, but you can feel it. I think it's a beautiful way to go through life and it's wonderful to share it with someone who believes the same.

After Susan's major surgery, I marvel at how she's bounced back. I see her doing things and think, *How does she keep going?* But then I remember the strength she showed raising two very sick boys and a daughter all those years while I was often away playing ball. She was and still is a powerful woman and a great mother. But sadly, for some time now, Kirstin has been our prodigal daughter. We've had some issues in recent years that may have stemmed from all the time we needed to give our sons under the direst of circumstances. We were so happy she was healthy and tried to do all we could for her, but life was still a challenge for all of us. As a result, we've had a falling out. As parents, it hurts because you're only as happy as your most unhappy child. And right now, we only have one. But we love Kirstin. She's our daughter and always will be.

It's normal for people to believe that the life of a professional ballplayer is a utopian existence with all the fame, fortune, and adulation we receive. And I was fortunate enough to have a lifetime of wonderful memories in baseball. But through all the high points, as my life demonstrates, we also deal with the same struggles, heartbreak, and obstacles as everyone else.

Life is hard. But with everything, I believe God is in control. And I'm taking things day by day.

ACKNOWLEDGMENTS

D WIGHT AND I WOULD LIKE TO GIVE SPECIAL THANKS to the following for their time and contributions to this book.

Red Sox teammates Carl Yastrzemski, Jim Rice, Fred Lynn, Bill Lee, Bruce Hurst, and Marty Barrett; baseball columnist and author Peter Gammons; and Red Sox broadcaster Joe Castiglione all gave valuable reflections, anecdotes, and insight into Dewey's career both on and off the field.

Sam Kennedy, the Red Sox president and CEO, for his recommendations and enthusiasm for the project.

Pam Kenn, the revered vice president of community, alumni, and player relations who is cherished by current and former Red Sox players alike for her meticulous work on their behalf, was a tremendous help in connecting me with team personnel and resources throughout this entire book project.

The Red Sox media relations department, with director Abby Murphy and coordinator Raleigh Clark, provided necessary access for my interviews at Fenway Park. And down on the farm, the senior vice president of the Worcester Red Sox, Brooke Cooper, graciously delivered on my requests concerning photos and information.

Karen Peluso, the longtime executive director of Neurofibromatosis Northeast, shared some of her wealth of knowledge about NF that will hopefully spread greater awareness of this devastating disease throughout these pages. And Suzanne Fountain, the associate vice president of the Jimmy Fund, provided anecdotal information on how Red Sox players have participated with the organization over the years to visit children afflicted by cancer.

The staff at the National Baseball Hall of Fame and Museum—led by Bruce Markusen, manager of digital and outreach learning, and Cassidy Lent, reference librarian in the Giamatti Research Center—was a tremendous help in providing me with files and press clippings from Dwight's playing career that proved extremely valuable to the project.

The team at Triumph Books, with whom I've written two other books, was once again a pleasure to work with. From publisher Noah Amstadter to senior acquisitions editor Josh Williams to senior editor Michelle Bruton, they all believed in this project right from the start. Their vision and enthusiasm for Dewey's remarkable story helped make it the inspiring book it became.

If there was a Hall of Fame for sports literary agents, Rob Wilson would certainly get my vote. As a former professional baseball player and editor for many years, there isn't another living soul in the publishing industry I would rather have as representation. His input, support, and advice benefitted the authors and this project in the most positive way.

I would also like to give recognition to various publications that helped in my research of Dewey's remarkable career. They include *Beyond the Sixth Game* by Peter Gammons, *Two Sides of Glory: The 1986 Boston Red Sox in Their Own Words* by Erik Sherman, *Boston Globe, Boston Herald, Providence Journal, Patriot Ledger, Los Angeles Times, New York Post, USA Today, Baltimore Sun, Times Union, National Sports Daily, Sports Illustrated, Sporting News, Sport Magazine, Inside Sports, 1975 Red Sox Program, 1975 Street and Smith's Official Baseball Yearbook,* and the *1976 Boston Red Sox Yearbook.*

Websites included Boston.com, HardballTimes.com, EagleTribune.com, Wikipedia.org, and the bible of baseball information BaseballReference.com. Information services and sources included the Elias Sports Bureau, United Press International, and the Associated Press.

And last, but certainly not least, Dwight and I would like to thank our wives, Susan Evans and Habiba Boumlik, for sacrificing significant spousal time so the extraordinary story of Dewey's life could be written.

—E.S.